KETO DIET

Ketogenic and Vegan Body

Author
Jenny A. Justice

Legal & Disclaimer

The information contained in this book and its contents is not designed to replace or take the place of any form of medical or professional advice; and is not meant to replace the need for independent medical, financial, legal or other professional advice or services, as may be required. The content and information in this book have been provided for educational and entertainment purposes only. The content and information contained in this book has been compiled from sources deemed reliable, and it is accurate to the best of the Author's knowledge, information and belief. However, the Author cannot guarantee its accuracy and validity and cannot be held liable for any errors and/or omissions. Further, changes are periodically made to this book as and when needed. Where appropriate and/or necessary, you must consult a professional (including but not limited to your doctor, attorney, financial advisor or such other professional advisor) before using any of the suggested remedies, techniques, or information in this book.

Upon using the contents and information contained in this book, you agree to hold harmless the Author from and against any damages, costs, and expenses, including any legal fees potentially resulting from the application of any of the information provided by this book. This disclaimer applies to any loss, damages or injury caused by the use and application, whether directly or indirectly, of any advice or information presented, whether for breach of contract, tort, negligence, personal injury, criminal intent, or under any other cause of action.

You agree to accept all risks of using the information presented inside this book.

You agree that by continuing to read this book, where appropriate and/or necessary, you shall consult a professional (including but not limited to your doctor, attorney, or financial advisor or such other advisor as needed) before using any of the suggested remedies, techniques, or information in this book.

Table of Contents

Introduction

Veganism is fast catching up with many people across the world. The noble idea behind veganism, such as not wanting to exploit the less fortunate animal species of the world by taking what is theirs and selfishly using it for ourselves simply because they do not have the power to stop us, is perhaps, the primary reason for the growth in popularity of this concept. However, in addition to the above extremely thoughtful reason, the health benefits and other great things about veganism are all sufficiently powerful causes for the expansion of the idea of veganism across the planet. This book is written with an intention to exhort newcomers to try a one-month vegan challenge that has the power to change not just your lifestyle but your entire outlook on life. Before you decide to try to change your lifestyle to vegan, there are a few things you must know and understand about it. This book aims to do exactly that by giving you a detailed overview in the following areas:

- What is veganism?
- A brief history on veganism
- How is veganism useful to you?
- Meal plans for a one-month challenge along with recipe outlines
- How to stay committed to the cause?

What is veganism?

You know who vegetarians are? They do not consume poultry, meat, or fish in their diet. Vegans, additionally, do not consume or use any animal products and/or by-products such as dairy products, honey, eggs, leather, silk, fur, and soaps and cosmetics made from animal sources. Vegans are the superset of vegetarians. All vegans are also vegetarians but all vegetarians need not be vegans.

Vegans believe that veganism is not just about their diet but a way of life. As far as possible, vegans avoid exploitation of animals in any form including but not limited to food, clothing, or other purposes. They also avoid items that have been tested on animals before being commercialized. And believe it or not, there is a vegan diet for all kinds of diets ranging from the junk food lovers to the raw food lovers and those in between, too.

History of Veganism

Veganism, although not known as veganism, has been around for many centuries. Examples of prevention of exploitation against and cruelty to animals have been written in history books. Lord Buddha of India and Pythagoras both advocated this concept and had put in rules to ensure their followers ate only plant-based food and completely avoided meats and animal products.

The earliest modern-day veganism is known to have occurred around 1806 CE. During that time, the great English poet P. B. Shelley and Dr. William Lambe publicly objected to consuming dairy products and eggs by humans on ethical grounds. This incident seems to have laid the foundation for modern-day veganism.

In November 1944, six non-dairy vegetarians including Donald Watson and Elsie Shrigley met together and discussed the topic on non-dairy vegetarians' lifestyles and diets. Despite strong opposition, these six members founded the new movement and became actively involved in this new project.

This book deals only with the dietary aspect of veganism, giving you ample sufficient reasons to shift your lifestyle to this healthy and noble one. While the benefits of turning vegan are discussed in another chapter, the kind of foods that you can include in your diet while keeping your energy levels and health not just unchanged but also improved than earlier is huge. Here is a small list of foods that are known to be totally vegan:

- *All kinds of grains and cereals*
- *All kinds of beans and legumes*
- *All fruits and vegetables*

Other vegan foods include soy milk, vegan mayonnaise, vegan ice cream and cheese, vegan hot dogs, and more. Moreover, a lot of companies have come out with mock meats that give vegans a sense of eating meat. This book also has four chapters dedicated to making vegan foods, which includes easy-to-make recipes.

Why Go Vegan?

Most people in the world want to do the following things by some means or the other:

- Lose weight
- Eat better
- Get fitter and healthier
- Do something for society and the world at large

The great news is that if you shift to a vegan diet, you can achieve all the above goals. And let me assure you, you will enjoy delicious, wholesome, and satiating meals as well.

No loss or reduction in energy levels – There is a misconception that changing to a vegan diet reduces your energy levels. There are numerous unworthy talks of vegans living only on water and a few greens and hence their energy levels have taken a huge dip. And on the other side of the spectrum, there are plenty of spurious rumors that say going vegan is helping them do impossible things. These other-end-of-the-spectrum talks make out vegans to be people who can walk on water! Let me assure you that neither of the extremes is true or based on any scientific studies.

Health benefits are huge when you choose to go vegan. Of course, the initial learning curve is going to be steep and you would have to counter multiple challenges. However, once you have overcome these tough phases and complete the 30-day challenge, you are going feel to happier, lighter, and fit. Moreover, there are multiple studies done by various organizations including the British Dietetic Association that has proven the excellent efficacies of getting fitter and healthier by following a vegan diet.

Here is the list of a few magic foods that can restore energy instantaneously:

Bananas – Already beautifully and naturally packaged by nature, this wonderful tropical fruit is normally the first you must reach out for when you feel tired or fatigued.

Walnuts – Another great pick-me-up tree nut, walnuts are rich in plant proteins, omega fatty acids, and vitamins giving you the almost-instant energy boost.

Green smoothies – Delicious smoothies made by tossing together strawberries, bananas, and orange juices are great and extremely healthy pick-me-ups to fight fatigue.

Coconut water – This is nature's energy drink and is amazingly refreshing and is filled with vitamins and potassium.

Kiwi – This low-fat delicious fruit is an instant energy enhancer triggered by the simple sugars present in it.

Why I chose to mention vegan energy boosters in the beginning itself is to help you overcome doubts regarding your ability to get on with your daily schedule if you choose to go vegan. Today there are many sportspeople who have shifted to this diet to keep fitter and sustain energy levels. So, if highly active people in the field of sports can take advantage of veganism, it should not be difficult for moderately active people like us to take this 30day challenge and come out with flying colors.

Other great reasons to take the one-month challenge to go vegan are:

Lose weight and yet remain energized – Many of us would love to find a sensible way to lose excess weight and yet remain healthy and fit. Average vegans are known to weigh 20 pounds lesser than average meateaters. Despite this, vegan diets do not starve you and make you feel enervated like the usual run-of-the-meal fad diets do.

Keep diseases and health disorders away – The Academy of Nutrition and Dietetics have conducted multiple studies which show that taking the vegan route helps you steer clear of common disorders such as diabetes, hypertension or high blood pressure thereby preventing the onset of many modern-day diseases such as heart attacks, kidney failure, and others.

Vegan foods are yummy and delicious – If you thought going vegan means you would have to give up your favorite ice creams, hamburgers, and chicken sandwiches, then you are wrong. With demand for vegan products soaring, many companies are coming up with amazingly delicious vegan options that taste very much like the non-vegetarian stuff. You will not miss any of the meats and animal products at all. There are plenty of established brands that cater to veganism and deliver really tasty dairy and meat substitutes.

Vegan diets are full of highly nutritious and healthy food items including whole grains, beans and legumes, nuts, soy products, and fresh fruits and vegetables. Here are some of the health benefits that these fiber-rich and healthy food sources provide you with:

- **Minimal saturated fats** – Meats and dairy products contain plenty of saturated fats thereby increasing the risk of cardiovascular diseases. Vegan diets automatically reduce intake of saturated fats enhancing your health condition

- **Fiber** – A vegan diet is high in fiber content that is very conducive to healthy bowel movements.

- **Magnesium** – Dark, green leafy vegetables are a rich source of magnesium, a key element that aids the body in the absorption of calcium.

- **Potassium** – Similarly, potassium, an important mineral that balances acidity and water in our body and helps in the removal of toxins, is found plenty in plant-based foods.

- **Proteins** – Meat-eaters invariably end up with more proteins than is needed by the body. Vegan diets, which include nuts, beans, and legumes, have the right amount of proteins for us.

Vegan diets provide other critically essential nutrients such as Vitamins E and C, phytochemicals, antioxidants, and foliate. These help in keeping your immunity system healthy and robust, and also prevent age-related diseases such as Alzheimer's and Parkinson's disease and keep your overall body organs functioning well.

Vegan diets have the power to prevent the following diseases that are very common in today's high-stress unhealthy lifestyle:

- Cardiovascular diseases

- Reduced cholesterol due to the complete absence of meat and dairy products in your diet

- Age-related macular degeneration

- Reduced risk of breast cancer

- Reduced risk of contracting ailments like diabetes, hypertension, cataracts, colon and prostate cancer, arthritis, and osteoporosis

In addition to improved health and prevention of diseases, going vegan makes you stronger, more energetic, and more attractive. Here is how: **Lowered Body Mass Index** – Cutting meat and dairy out of your diet naturally reduces Body Mass Index.

Weight loss – Weight loss is an unquestioned effect of a vegan diet.

Healthy skin – Consuming rich sources of Vitamins A and E from nuts and fruits and vegetables enhance the texture and health of your skin.

Reduced allergy symptoms – Plant-based foods do not trigger as many allergic reactions in humans as dairy and meat products do.

Less intake of mercury – A lot of shellfish and fish contain high levels of mercury, which we take in when we eat these foods. Switching to veganism does away with this toxin completely.

The above are only some of the great reasons that you must start off this 30day vegan challenge. Instead of finding reasons not to do something good, focus on the above reasons which tell you why you should do it and dive straight in. Summon some extra willpower and after you complete this challenge you can rest assured that the willpower would come on its own when you see and feel the wondrous new VEGAN YOU.

Chapter 1: What is a Ketogenic Vegan Diet

Before you dive into a new diet, you should always make sure that you know what that diet is and what it entails. So, first things first. What is a ketogenic diet? A ketogenic diet is categorized as a diet, this being very low carb but very high fat. This is not the first time most people are hearing this as they've heard about other diets of this sort as well. While this diet can be similar to others, there are also differences that set it apart. What this diet is designed to do is it puts your body into a state called ketosis. This is a metabolic state that is a reduction of carbs and it means you're reducing how much your intake of carbs is and instead, you're replacing it with fat. They believe that when you adopt this diet, your body will become more efficient at burning your fat and turning it into energy. It's also believed that the fats in your liver will turn into ketones. After they turn to ketones, it is said by some that your brain will now have more energy because of this process.

As with a vegetarian diet, there are people who classify themselves as a different type of ketogenic. While there is a debate on which is the best, there are four that are most commonly chosen among people.
The high protein ketogenic diet, which has things in common with a standard ketogenic diet (but as the title implies), has more protein than the standard version. The ratio is, of course, different as well. For a high protein ketogenic diet, you have thirty-five percent proteins, with sixty percent fat and only five percent is made up of carbs.

The targeted ketogenic diet is another ketogenic diet that a lot of people enjoy. This one is very similar to the others except that for this, a targeted ketogenic diet allows you to add carbs to your diet around workouts. This is actually one of two ketogenic diets on this list that allows you to change the number of carbs that you're allowed to use.

A cyclical ketogenic diet is a diet that uses the idea of Refeeding is the process of eating more calories than you have in previous days. People believe that the process of refeeding is beneficial in losing fat because it is supposed to boost metabolism and ideally stop you from falling into a calorie deficit or crashing. So, this diet will be using higher refeeds than the other forms of ketogenic diets on this list. This is the only one on this list that allows you to have cheat days. They believe that you should have two higher carb days and five ketogenic days. They also stress that the two carb days should follow the ketogenic days and not before.

Finally, we come to the standard ketogenic diet. This is the most popular of the four and most people choose this diet as their go-to for this lifestyle. The standard diet believes that you should have only twenty percent protein and five percent carbs but have a seventy-five percent allowance for your fat. It is most assuredly a high-fat diet with extremely low carbs but still maintaining moderate protein. The thing to remember here is low carb. There are many vegan foods that you shouldn’t eat on a ketogenic diet like pasta, tortillas, bread, pretzels and other snack foods like chips or crackers, soda, cereal, fruit juices, and most fruits. These are all too high in carbs for a ketogenic diet.

You’ll need to stay away from packaged foods with refined flour or sugar, rice, white potatoes, sweet potatoes, and starchy vegetables. There are still plenty of other items you can eat so if it seems like you’re really limited, you’re not. You just need to work around what you can’t eat.

Any of these diets would benefit you although obviously, as each diet has differences, you will need to determine which is going to help you the most because you know what your goals are.
Originally, a ketogenic diet was believed to be a helpful aid to help with epilepsy and seizures. One of the things that are stressed about this is that the ketogenic diet is very specialized since it needs to be done with the guidance, supervision, and care of trained medical specialists. In certain countries of the world, they will only offer adult treatment in very few clinics because more data and research are needed about the impact the diet will have on adults. Through careful monitoring with specialists, doctors, and nutritionists, they say there can be benefits for children with epilepsy and seizures using this diet, but they are still conducting more research on this as well.

Other studies have shown that the ketogenic diet may reduce symptoms of Parkinson's disease or polycystic ovary syndrome in women by reducing insulin levels. It has been debated in others that it may be used to treat different kinds of cancer or tumor growth or reduce symptoms of Alzheimer's disease or possibly slow down its progression. When scientists did a study on animals, they learned that on an animal brain, the diet could reduce concussions and help recovery after a brain injury but obviously, an animal's brain is vastly different than humans and we don't know if the same results would be reflected in a human brain.

It has been debated but, in some cases, people found that some of the test subjects lost two times more weight on the ketogenic diet than on a low-fat diet that restricts calories. Like veganism, which means that you don't consume any animal product at all whatsoever, a ketogenic diet is also said to help with type two diabetes. However, the ketogenic diet is said in one study to have improved insulin by seventy-five percent.

Another study even found that seven people out of the twenty-one participants were able to stop using their diabetic medication. Now, obviously, that doesn't mean it will happen for everyone as everyone's health and body can be different and some people may have had diabetes longer than others. That's why more research is needed on the subject so that we can have more concrete answers and evidence.

Possible Downsides to Having a Vegan Ketogenic Diet

One of the main reasons people become vegans is to help the animals as they feel its morally and ethically wrong to eat them because it's cruel and inhumane. They also have moral and ethical issues about how eating animals effects the planet. But believe it or not, while there are many benefits to being vegan and adopting a vegan ketogenic diet, there are also downsides not just for your health but for the planet as well.

The planet has many poor countries. Some so poor that they feed their children dirt before they go to school because it’s all their community has. Some so poor that they are dying without proper water. In some of these poor countries, they need all the meat they can get because they may not be able to nourish their people with anything else. The same situation is present in countries where grazing is efficient because they don’t have any land that is suitable for growing or sustaining crops.

Another reason it might not be the best is that if we all stop eating meat, the planet would be overpopulated with animals and then the emissions would grow higher because their still producing manure but now, there’s more of it and the wheat that could be feeding starving people is being used to feed animals instead. This sounds heartless and like the animals should be eaten for meat, which is not what I am saying at all. The animals deserve to live as any other creature. We are merely presenting facts.

Remember the countries that don’t have soil that can produce good crops? As people will be eating less meat, that means they will need to eat more plants. In those lands that have soil which won't produce, the sheep, cattle, and goats are actually helping make that inedible grass and turning it into edible milk and meat for the people. In some countries, that milk and meat is their only source of protein and fat to keep them nourished. If you take it away, what do they have left if they don't have crops?

Also, the land mostly used for nuts, fruits, and vegetables is cultivated cropland. Grazing cropland is usually unsuitable for attempting to grow crops but is actually really good at feeding animals that we use for food such as cattle. The last type of cropland that we have is called perennial cropland.

This is good for grain, hay, and other types of crops that are alive yearround. What they do is harvest these crops multiple times before dying. The reason the vegan diet sticks out here is that it's the only diet that doesn't use all of the lands. It specifically doesn't use perennial cropland which would waste the chance to produce more food for the people of the planet.

The livestock industry, though hated by some, also creates a livelihood or jobs and means of support for over one billion of the world's poor families and employs over one point three billion people. Without the livestock industry, those families would be out of a job.

The shocking thing about greenhouse gasses is that while most people believe that meat is causing many greenhouse emissions (and they are, believe it or not), it has been proven that some vegetables can cause just as many gasses as meat! Studies have shown that if you're going by calories, making lettuce can create as much greenhouse emissions as beef. It has been shown that lettuce generates about three times what pork or fresh fish does in greenhouse gasses. That's crazy, right?

Food waste is also a really big problem that takes a toll on the environment. Fruits and vegetables tend to be one of the highest wasted foods at forty percent to the only thirty-three percent that meat does. That's only a seven percent difference but it does add up. One issue that makes these findings difficult is that it also varies from country to country with what people throw away and waste. Some things are agreed upon though and it's what makes the science easier to comprehend. Perishability is also another argument. Fruits, vegetables, and a lot of other things that vegans need to survive perish very quickly and most people are more likely to throw away these food items than dairy or meat because they've gone bad. So, while a vegan world would benefit in many ways, it would also hurt in a few ways as well especially if it's not sustainable for many people because of where or how they live.

There are also health problems that can arise from you being a vegan and a ketogenic. We will start with the problems that arise from being a vegan first. Osteoporosis is a serious health issue that can arise if you're not eating properly. Calcium is a very important nutrient that you shouldn't ignore and yet, unfortunately, there are many in the vegan lifestyle that can do just that. This can cause your bones to become weak and result in fractures and damage you might not be able to repair at all. Ways to keep your calcium up as a vegetarian are to eat items like kale and Chinese cabbage or spinach and broccoli. High potassium items with high magnesium can reduce blood acidity. You can find items like this in the fruits and vegetables you would just need to check. Lowering the blood acidity is helpful because you are lowering the chances of excreting calcium through your urine.

Regardless of what you eat on this particular diet, you might still need a supplement if you're not getting the things you need for your body. For example, studies have shown that most vegans do not get enough vitamin D and may need to take a supplement to correct that. One nutrient that they will need a supplement for no matter what they eat is a vitamin B12 supplement since B12 is only found in animal products. Since this includes dairy products, vegans don't have the option of not taking one as vegetarians do, and they have no choice but to take a supplement to make sure they are getting the right amount in their body or it can be detrimental to their health. One of the biggest debates about the ketogenic diet is whether going into ketosis is safe. Ketosis can actually be dangerous when your ketones build up. It can lead to high levels of dehydration and it is said that it can change the chemical balance of your blood. Another problem is if ketosis goes too far, the body can go into ketoacidosis. This is what happens when ketones build up in your blood. When they build up in your blood, it becomes acidic. This can cause your body to go into ketoacidosis which can cause you to fall into a coma or die. People with diabetes are especially susceptible to ketoacidosis if they don't take enough insulin or if they're injured or sick. People can also fall into ketoacidosis when they have an overactive ethnocide or be caused by starvation.

It's very important to understand that if your feeling tired or have flushed skin, throwing up, confusion, pain in your stomach, fruity smelling breath, feeling thirsty or even urinating a lot, these are all signs of ketoacidosis and you should call a doctor right away. Especially when you have diabetes, the symptoms may start slowly with throwing up, but the process speeds up quickly in just a few hours. So, when you're in ketosis, you need to make sure you don't fall into ketoacidosis because it can lead to fatal sickness.

Lastly, another reason to be cautious is that in a ketogenic diet, your insulin levels begin to go down. This causes your body to shed water and sodium. When the body does it, this is beginning to do what is called reduced bloat. It can also cause dehydration and lightheadedness or constipation and headaches. Low sodium is bad for the body because if your sodium and electrolyte levels are low, you can have muscle weakness and changes in blood pressure. More scarily, your heartbeat can become irregular.

Dehydration is also a big issue with the ketogenic diet because, in the first two weeks, you're losing water and electrolytes. It's also known as a water flushing diet because there is a lessening of inflammation. There is also a reduction of glycogen stores in your liver and muscles. To keep yourself from getting dehydrated, you might need to drink about two liters or more a day. You should start when you begin cutting the carbs in your diet because of being ketogenic.

Social media is also dangerous on this diet or honestly any diet. Many people think they're helping or being supportive. Those people are alright as long as they're giving the proper advice. Others like tearing others down and giving bad advice. One big problem that many people encounter unfortunately is bad advice. If you go on social media, there are so many people trying to tell you how to live your life and how you should go about it. Now, to be fair, most of these people think that they are helping. Some of them are and they've done their research to make sure that they are giving good advice and they've talked to doctors to make sure that the information they are giving people is good information. Others, however, can be causing damage to people and making them sick. For example, one social media user says she only eats a certain number of calories a day. If you do your homework, you'll realize those are eating disorder levels and not healthy. As many young women and men watch her channel, this person could be potentially harming thousands of young people and they could think that eating disorders are alright when they are not. Eating disorders affect so many people these days. When you're dieting, it's so important to make sure you're taking in the proper calories so that you don't fall into dangerous territories. You will also need to eat a variety of foods. This prevents you from falling into other dangerous territories like orthorexia.

Others on social media say that you can eat over five thousand calories a day (most of which are certain types of sugar), not work out, and you will lose weight and not have health problems. That is simply untrue and that can be potentially life-threatening advice. Some people have diabetes and that much sugar can put them into ketoacidosis which can be fatal. The scary part about this is that for diabetics, it can become fatal in a matter of hours. That's a terrifying thought. Even normal people who don't have any issues can be severely damaged by this advice. You can gain weight which causes many health problems on its own; you cannot ingest that many calories and not work out and expect that you won't put on any pounds at all. You will because you're consuming so many calories a day. There are many other problems with this advice as well and people shouldn't follow extreme diets because it's not safe and it's misleading to give people advice without making sure that it's safe for the people who are listening to you.

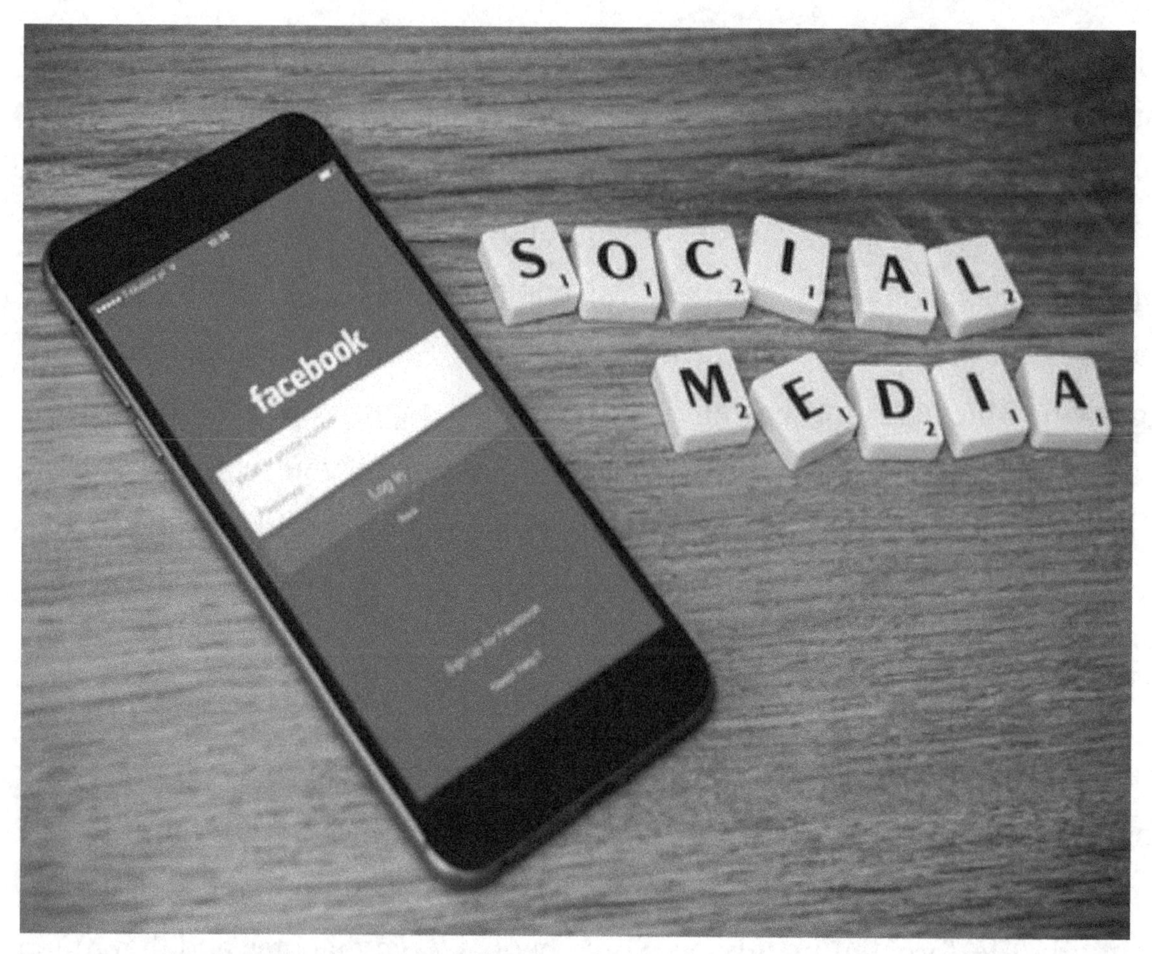

Everyone can get on social media these days. We live in a digital world and children and teenagers younger and younger are taking advice from the net and not their parents. This is not a good thing. There is so much information on the internet that isn't true and even more dangerous to impressionable young minds. People on the net or social media say that they can say what they want and shouldn't have to worry about what they say but they should. They are considered role models to people around the world and with a society so crazed about diets, we need to understand what real information that is the right information is and what is false and dangerous to our health. Fast food options for vegans are not the healthiest either and they're kind of difficult to come by sometimes. So, when going out into this diet, you'll need to be careful about where you go. If you live in certain areas where veganism is more prominent, then you'll probably have more access to vegan-friendly restraints. Whereas if you live somewhere where it's more meat inclined, not so much. In these cases, your supermarkets will probably also have a harder time having good vegan options as well which can be a pain.

If you do manage to find a vegan option at a fast-food restraint, you still need to remember your golden rule. Check the ingredients and know the calorie information as well as your micros and macros. Just because it is a vegan option doesn't mean that its ketogenic as well. You need to make sure that whatever you're going, go for the healthy option. Remember there are foods on this diet that you can eat but they're not healthy for your goals.

Most ketogenic also make what is called a fat bomb. This is a very popular trend in the Keto world, but it may not be the safest one. The 'fat bombs' are usually high in fat, of course, with a moderate amount of either artificial or natural sweetness. Keto dieters usually refer to fat bombs as a treat, snack, or dessert. Some use it before a workout.
Some use it as a fat dense snack or a way to curb their sweet tooth. With the Keto diet, you're trying to cut sugar and carbs. You're trying to eat cleaner. These fat bombs are usually ninety percent fat or even more. The fat from these bombs commonly comes from coconut milk or from dairy. While most use it as a snack or dessert, some actually use it for a meal replacement. There is so much fat in these bombs that the calories for a single one can be anywhere from two hundred and fifty calories to five hundred calories.

We know that Keto dieters strive for higher fat but depending on your calorie intake for the day, you're using a big chunk of your calories for a small little goodie.

The goal of the Keto diet is to achieve ketosis. When you reach for snacks like you would with a fat bomb, it could mean you're not in a state of ketosis any longer. Meaning, fat bombs are basically promoting snacking unnecessarily. Boiled eggs are a better way to respond to hunger. Your body needs to take its own time on this diet and there is no quick fix. If you suddenly begin to consume large amounts of fat, that's not going to make you adjust quicker.

The Keto diet's success is the result of hormones; one hormone in specific as a matter of fact. It's called leptin. Leptin reacting to a lack of blood sugar in your body results in your body using stored fat for energy. The fat that is consumed for the energy would be used before the stored fat. This means that the benefits of fat bombs are diminished in terms of fat loss. This is because while you could be maintaining ketosis, you're fueling your ketones with the wrong thing. You're fueling them with fat bombs instead of an extra arm, stomach, or thigh fat.

Insulin and leptin are opposing hormones in your body. One tells the body to stop storing fat, the other tells the body to store fat. Many people are concerned with insulin and insulin resistance. But a higher priority needs to be given to leptin. In the human body, any hormone that you overproduce decreases the body's sensitivity to it. So in a body that has excess fat, the hormone leptin is being overused. The impact of leptin resistance in the body is that the body does not know how or when to stop storing fat. So the fat could come from frying oil or coconut oil, but it wouldn't matter.

Another thing nutritionist say is that if you want to slim down, a ketogenic diet is not the best way to do this. It's considered extreme and nutritionists warn it may not be healthy. Others say that it's not sustainable for people and they believe it's just not a good diet for you. Since this diet is also low in fiber, it's been said that that can cause digestive issues with your body. They believe if you do a more balanced diet, it will be better for your future diets and goal

Chapter 2 Eating Healthy

If you haven't already been tracking your "macros and micros" for your regular vegan diet, it's about time that you started. There is no better way to make sure you're getting the exact amount of calories, and the exact amount of nutrients, that your body needs without tracking your macros and micros.

"Macros" is an abbreviation that stands for "macronutrients," and they're what the Keto diet is based on. The three main macronutrients required for human life are carbohydrates, proteins, and fats. That's right! Tracking your macronutrients is just as easy as tracking how many grams of protein, carbohydrates, and fats you're eating in each meal. It does get a bit more complicated than that, but it's nothing you won't be able to handle. "Micros," then, stands for "micronutrients," and these are quite different from what you might be thinking.

Micronutrients are actually the vitamins and minerals that your body requires to function, and micros are often essential for macros to do their jobs. Without the help of certain minerals, our macronutrients wouldn't be able to synthesize new proteins, add in our cellular regeneration, and help move bad molecules like harmful cholesterol out of our arteries. In order to make sure you're getting your proper dosages of micronutrients, you take supplements! One of the many helpful connections between veganism and the Keto diet is that both tend to require a healthy amount of added vitamins and minerals. Check back to **Chapter 1** if you need a refresher.

However, it's worth noting that there are many more suggested micronutrients that we're supposed to get per day beyond just the popular five or seven. In fact, there are a whopping twenty-five micronutrients that our diets are supposed to provide us with every day. Although some of the amounts are so small, they're measured in micrograms—it's worth taking a look at this list to know what else you might want to supplement.

A multivitamin in combination with your regular vegan diet supplements should supply you with the perfect amount of each of these smaller micronutrients. You should, however, consult your physician before you start taking iron supplements. Tracking your macronutrients is definitely more involved, but there's a special tool that we're going to borrow from the body-building community to make it easier.

How Weighing Your Portions Ensures Success:

Nobody likes a scale, but isn't it true that everything's better when there's food involved? Back when the fitness community began to really focus on how our diets were facilitating weight loss, many body-builders and intense athletes started to use food scales as a way to be more precise about the portion sizes. But not just portions of whole meals—weighing your food with a food scale allows you to calculate the number of macronutrients **and** the number of calories in each portion of the meals you're going to prepare each week. The first step to using your food scale is to download an app called MyFitnessPal (the most popular macronutrient tracking app out there, and a great community to get involved with if you're vegan!).

If you don't have a smartphone, feel free to use an online calculator—you'll be able to find more than a few. The next step is to visit your local restaurant supply store to stock up on large containers. Each week, when you prepare your meal on Sunday, you'll want to use your food scale to weight the entire cooked meal (all three or four portions together). To do this, set your chosen container on your scale and make the numbers read "00.00" – you're going to be pouring your entire meal into these containers to measure, so bigger is better. Once you've measured the full meal, use your application to plug in each of the ingredients you used in the meal and their amounts.

This is just another reason that it's important to be organized with your grocery shopping. The resulting numbers should give you the number of total calories and nutrients, and if you divide by the number of portions you intend for the meal to make, you'll have an accurate nutritional label of calories, vitamins, and nutrients.

Prepare to Meal Prep

Meal prep, short for meal preparation, is a technique known far and wide in the fitness community as one of the best ways to ensure that you're eating a protein-packed, well-balanced meal with the proper portions to maximize your weight loss (or gain) without taking up too much time. During the week, most of us work forty hours or more—and if you're adding in the time that it takes to go to the gym, commute back and forth, finish your weekly work, and manage whatever other responsibilities you have—there isn't much time left for home-cooking. However, the meals you might purchase at a supermarket or restaurant simply won't fit in with a strict diet, especially one that combines two strict methods of eating. Meal prep is a great technique for busy individuals to use to make sure that they're getting the proper amount of fats, proteins, and carbohydrates for their diet and fitness.

When you're eating a vegan Keto diet, you want to pay extra attention to the breakdown of nutrients in your food (and how those nutrients measure up in terms of carbohydrate content). Skip down to the section titled "Meal Prep Tips for Vegans Eating Keto" to get a better handle on your nutrient breakdown if you're already familiar with how to meal prep. If you aren't, everything you need to know is right below.

How to Meal Prep

The idea behind meal prepping is incredibly simple, but the timing is a little less self-explanatory. Meal prepping is a practice that takes place normally on a Sunday before the work week begins when most people have enough time to cook multiple large-batch meals in one day. Yes, you'll most likely end up cooking more meals on Sunday than you'll get to eat. It's alright. You'll thank yourself late in the week. Meal prepping on Sundays normally starts with a trip to the grocery store to make sure your produce is as fresh as possible. While some more advanced meal prep specialists have adapted to using their freezer for fresh ingredients, you'll only want to rely on your freezer for full meals at the beginning of your journey.

Normally meal prep consists of all the dinner, lunches, breakfasts, and snacks you can possibly prepare to give yourself time to go to the gym and get enough sleep while you're working. The easiest way to tackle meal prep for the first time is to start by making four lunches and four dinners in one Sunday. Although that might seem like a fair amount, it's really only two meals that you'll be cooking in large batches. Meal prep is known for creating quite the large mess in the kitchen, so take the time to do a bit of pre-cleaning so that you won't regret it afterward. A pre-clean is a great time to make sure all your largest pots, saucepans, and skillets and ready to cook with; one meal might not always mean one pot.

Many vegan Keto recipes rely on sautéing, steaming, and grilling in order to give a smoky depth of flavor to foods with a more neutral palette. While your gathering your cooking utensils, remember that meal prepping is all about organization. Before you go to the grocery store, make sure you have all your ingredients written down and that you know what to look for when it comes to labels. High carb content in both carbs and **net** carbs will impact your ability to reach Ketosis. Once you're ready to start cooking, make sure you have plenty of healthy cooking oils on hand to lubricate your pans.

Coconut oil is recommended, but with its low smoke point, you're welcome to use olive oil if you need to cook hotter for longer. After you're finished, it's crucial that you have equal sized Tupperware for proper storage. Nothing ruins a good middle of the week meal like opening your squash spaghetti to freezer burn. Most cooked meals take three to five days to go bad, so while you don't have to put your prepped meals in the freezer, sometimes it's a good back up if your fridge is low on space. That's about all there is to the process of preparing your meals, but what about prepping meals specifically for a vegan Keto diet? Does anything change?

Meal Prep Tips for Vegans Eating Keto

A vegan Keto diet isn't the **most** restrictive diet out there, but it's certainly one of the more admirable challenges in the health and fitness world. Sticking to a vegan Keto diet can be hard, but meal prepping the best vegan Keto meals will make a world of difference when it comes to upholding your commitment. Many of our lives are constantly busy, and when you're trying to maintain a Keto diet, it's imperative that you eat at the same time each day—especially if you're on a fast. This might mean eating at work or packing a meal to take with you for after the gym. Either way, preparing your necessary meals each week will give you more time to focus on your mental health and less time worrying about pounds that will melt off naturally.

You'll also be able to portion out your carbs, fats, and proteins according to your Keto guidelines, which will help infinitely in organizing. As a vegan eating Keto, you'll also want to make sure that you're paying special attention to things like generated plastic waste—if you're trying to save the planet by eating less meat, it doesn't make much sense to package your snacks each day in disposable Ziploc baggies. Glass Tupperware are the cornerstones of vegan meal prep containers, and the many different sizes and tight lids of Mason jars are perfect for taking your snacks and salads on the go. But meal preparation is more than just saving you time, money, and precious calories.

Portioning out your meals is a key part of both veganism and the Keto diet because of your need to more urgently check certain nutrition boxes. These nutrition boxes are called you macronutrients and micronutrients, and if fats, carbs, and proteins thought they were the only reason we portioned out or meals, they were very wrong. Tracking your "macros and micros" is just like making sure you don't eat too much bread in one day—except for your body, it's a lot more serious. These essential chemicals can sometimes mean the difference between a perfectly healthy body, and one that struggles to function

Chapter 3 Cooking Tips for Beans, Legumes, and Grains

1. Soak beans for at least 8 to 10 hours (preferably overnight) to remove any anti-nutrients. This reduces the chances of stomach cramps, gas, and bloating.
2. If you're pressed for time, you can also use a quick **Soak Method**. Just boil enough water to cover the beans, add in the beans, let simmer for 10 minutes, and set aside for an hour.
3. Soak quinoa and brown rice for a couple of hours. Lentils and other grains don't require any prior soaking.

Cooking utensils

1. Cooking in a pressure cooker

Drain the water from one cup of previously soaked beans, grains, or lentils. Rinse the vegetables well and add them to a 6-to 8-quart cooker.
Add 2-4 cups of water. Close the lid and cook on high heat.
When the cooker reaches a high pressure, lower the heat, and cook for an extra 7-10 minutes. Turn off the heat, let everything cool, and open the lid.

2. Cooking in a slow cooker

Drain the water from one cup of previously soaked beans/quinoa/brown rice, rinse well, and add to a smaller slow cooker.
Pour in 2-4 cups of water. Add other ingredients except for salt (for stews, soups, and one pot meals). Cover the slow cooker with a lid and cook on high heat for 3-4 hours, or 7-8 hours on low heat. Add in salt in the last 10 minutes of cooking.

3. *Cooking Grains and Lentils on a Stovetop*

Respect the following quantities when cooking on a stove top. Water and Yield are measured in cups, and time in minutes.

Chapter 4 Vigan Recipes

Breakfast

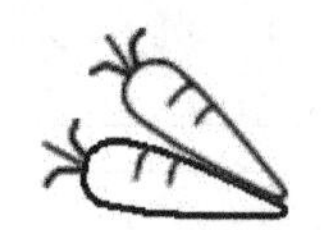

1 Keto Porridge

Total Time: 10 minutes Serves: 1

½ tsp. vanilla extract
¼ tsp. granulated stevia
1 tbsp. chia seeds
1 tbsp. flaxseed meal
2 tbsp. unsweetened shredded coconut
2 tbsp. almond flour
2 tbsp. hemp hearts
½ cup water
Pinch of salt
Add all ingredients except vanilla extract to a saucepan and heat over low heat until thickened. Stir well and serve warm.

Nutritional Value (Amount per Serving): Calories 370; Fat 30.2 g; Carbohydrates 12.8 g; Sugar 1.9 g; Protein 13.5 g; Cholesterol 0 mg

2 Easy Chia Seed Pudding

Total Time: 10 minutes Serves: 4

¼ tsp. cinnamon
15 drops liquid stevia
½ tsp. vanilla extract
½ cup chia seeds
2 cups unsweetened coconut milk
Add all ingredients into the glass jar and mix well.
Close jar with lid and place in refrigerator for 4 hours.
Serve chilled and enjoy.

Nutritional Value (Amount per Serving): Calories 347; Fat 33.2 g; Carbohydrates 9.8 g; Sugar 4.1 g; Protein 5.9 g; Cholesterol 0 mg

3 Delicious Vegan Zoodles

Total Time: 15 minutes Serves: 4

4 small zucchinis, spiralized into noodles
3 tbsp vegetable stock
1 cup red pepper, diced
1/2 cup onion, diced
3/4 cup nutritional yeast
1 tbsp garlic powder
Pepper
Salt
Add zucchini noodles, red pepper, and onion in a pan with vegetable stock and cook over medium heat for few minutes.
Add nutritional yeast and garlic powder and cook for few minutes until creamy.
Season with pepper and salt.
Stir well and serve.

Nutritional Value (Amount per Serving): Calories 71; Fat 0.9 g; Carbohydrates 12.1 g; Sugar 5.7 g; Protein 5.7 g; Cholesterol 0 mg

4 Avocado Tofu Scramble

Total Time: 15 minutes Serves: 1

1 tbsp fresh parsley, chopped
½ medium avocado
½ block firm tofu, drained and crumbled
½ cup bell pepper, chopped
½ cup onion, chopped
1 tsp olive oil

1 tbsp water
¼ tsp cumin
¼ tsp garlic powder
¼ tsp paprika
¼ tsp turmeric
1 tbsp nutritional yeast
Pepper
Salt

In a bowl, mix together nut yeast, water, and spices. Put separately Now heat the olive oil to the pan over medium heat.
Add onion and bell pepper and sauté for 5 minutes.
Add crumbled tofu and nutritional yeast to the pan and sauté for 2 minutes.
Top with parsley and avocado.
Serve and enjoy.

Nutritional Value (Amount per Serving): Calories 164; Fat 9.7 g; Carbohydrates 15 g; Sugar 6 g; Protein 7.4 g; Cholesterol 0 mg

5 Delicious Tofu Fries

Total Time: 50 minutes Serves: 4

15 oz firm tofu, drained, pressed and cut into long strips
¼ tsp garlic powder
¼ tsp onion powder
¼ tsp cayenne pepper
¼ tsp paprika
½ tsp oregano

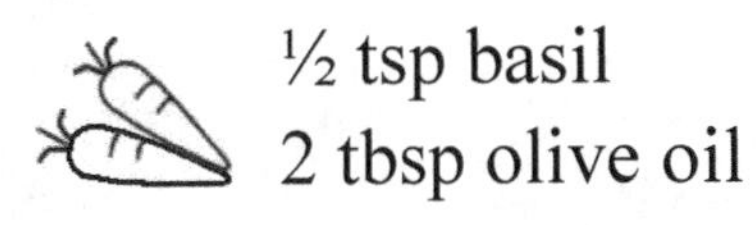

½ tsp basil
2 tbsp olive oil
Pepper
Salt

Preheat the oven to 190 C/ 375 F.
Add all ingredients into the large mixing bowl and toss well.
Place marinated tofu strips on a baking tray and bake in preheated oven for 20 minutes.
Turn tofu strips to other side and bake for another 20 minutes. Serve and enjoy.

Nutritional Value (Amount per Serving): Calories 137; Fat 11.5 g; Carbohydrates 2.3 g; Sugar 0.8 g; Protein 8.8 g; Cholesterol 0 mg

6 Chia Raspberry Pudding Shots

Total Time: 10 minutes Serves: 4

½ cup raspberries
10 drops liquid stevia
1 tbsp unsweetened cocoa powder
¼ cup unsweetened almond milk
½ cup unsweetened coconut milk
¼ cup chia seeds
Add all ingredients into the glass jar and stir well to combine.
Pour pudding mixture into the shot glasses and place in refrigerator for 1 hour.
Serve chilled and enjoy.

Nutritional Value (Amount per Serving): Calories 117; Fat 10 g; Carbohydrates 5.9 g; Sugar 1.7 g; Protein 2.7 g; Cholesterol 0 mg

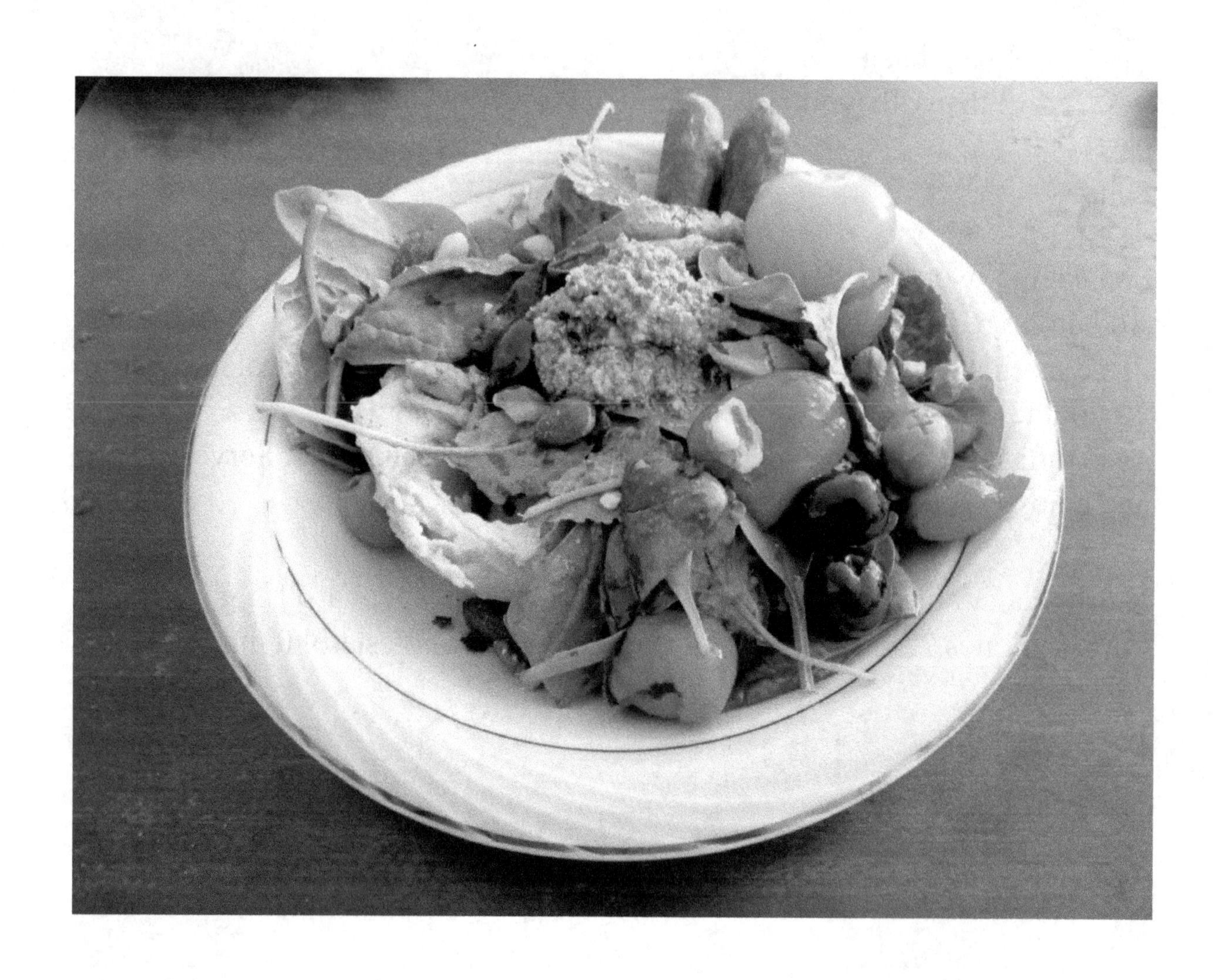

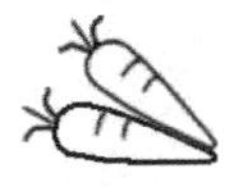

7 Healthy Chia-Almond Pudding

Total Time: 10 minutes Serves: 2

½ tsp vanilla extract
¼ tsp almond extract
2 tbsp ground almonds
1 ½ cups unsweetened almond milk ¼
cup chia seeds

Add chia seeds in almond milk and soak for 1 hour.
Add chia seed and almond milk into the blender.
Add remaining ingredients to the blender and blend until smooth and creamy. Serve and enjoy.

Nutritional Value (Amount per Serving): Calories 138; Fat 10.2 g; Carbohydrates 6 g; Sugar 0.5 g; Protein 5.1 g; Cholesterol 0 mg

8 Fresh Berries with Cream

Total Time: 10 minutes Serves: 1

1/2 cup coconut cream
1 oz strawberries
1 oz raspberries
1/4 tsp vanilla extract

Add all ingredients into the blender and blend until smooth.
Pour in serving bowl and top with fresh berries.
Serve and enjoy.

Nutritional Value (Amount per Serving): Calories 303; Fat 28.9 g; Carbohydrates 12 g; Sugar 6.8 g; Protein 3.3 g; Cholesterol 0 mg

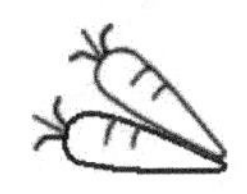

9 Almond Hemp Heart Porridge

Total Time: 10 minutes Serves: 2

¼ cup almond flour
½ tsp cinnamon
¾ tsp vanilla extract
5 drops stevia
1 tbsp chia seeds
2 tbsp ground flax seed
½ cup hemp hearts
1 cup unsweetened coconut milk

Add all ingredients except almond flour to a saucepan. Stir to combine.
Heat over medium heat until just starts to lightly boil.
Once start bubbling then stir well and cook for 1 minute more.
Remove from heat and stir in almond flour.
Serve immediately and enjoy.

Nutritional Value (Amount per Serving): Calories 329; Fat 24.4 g; Carbohydrates 9.2 g; Sugar 1.8 g; Protein 16.2 g; Cholesterol 0 mg

10 Cauliflower Zucchini Fritters

Total Time: 15 minutes Serves: 4

3 cups cauliflower florets

¼ tsp black pepper
¼ cup coconut flour
2 medium zucchini, grated and squeezed
1 tbsp coconut oil
½ tsp sea salt

Steam cauliflower florets for 5 minutes.
Add cauliflower into the food processor and process until it looks like rice.
Add all ingredients except coconut oil to the large bowl and mix until well combined.
Make small round patties from the mixture and set aside.
Heat coconut oil in a pan over medium heat.
Place patties on pan and cook for 3-4 minutes on each side.
Serve and enjoy.

Nutritional Value (Amount per Serving): Calories 68; Fat 3.8 g; Carbohydrates 7.8 g; Sugar 3.6 g; Protein 2.8 g; Cholesterol 0 mg

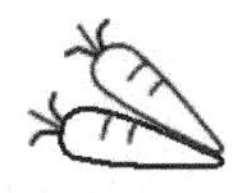

11 Chocolate Strawberry Milkshake

Total Time: 5 minutes Serves: 2

1 cup ice cubes
¼ cup unsweetened cocoa powder
2 scoops vegan protein powder
1 cup strawberries
2 cups unsweetened coconut milk

Add all ingredients into the blender and blend until smooth and creamy. Serve immediately and enjoy.

Nutritional Value (Amount per Serving): Calories 221; Fat 5.7 g; Carbohydrates 15 g; Sugar 6.8 g; Protein 27.7 g; Cholesterol 0 mg

12 Coconut Blackberry Breakfast Bowl

Total Time: 10 minutes Serves: 2

2 tbsp chia seeds
¼ cup coconut flakes
1 cup spinach
¼ cup water
3 tbsp ground flaxseed
1 cup unsweetened coconut milk

1 cup blackberries

Add blackberries, flaxseed, spinach, and coconut milk into the blender and blend until smooth.

Fry coconut flakes in pan for 1-2 minutes.

Pour berry mixture into the serving bowls and sprinkle coconut flakes and chia seeds on top.

Serve immediately and enjoy.

Nutritional Value (Amount per Serving): Calories 182; Fat 11.4 g; Carbohydrates 14.5 g; Sugar 4.3 g; Protein 5.3 g; Cholesterol 0 mg

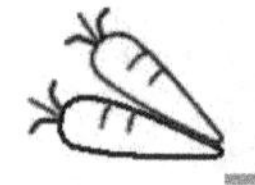

13 Cinnamon Coconut Pancake

Total Time: 15 minutes Serves: 1

1/2 cup almond milk
1/4 cup coconut flour
2 tbsp egg replacer
8 tbsp water
1 packet stevia
1/8 tsp cinnamon
1/2 tsp baking powder
1 tsp vanilla extract
1/8 tsp salt

In a small bowl, mix together egg replacer and 8 tablespoons of water.

Add all ingredients into the mixing bowl and stir until combined.

Spray pan with cooking spray and heat over medium heat.
Pour the desired amount of batter onto hot pan and cook until lightly golden brown.
Flip pancake and cook for a few minutes more.
Serve and enjoy.

Nutritional Value (Amount per Serving): Calories 110; Fat 4.3 g; Carbohydrates 10.9 g; Sugar 2.8 g; Protein 7 g; Cholesterol 0 mg

14 Flax Almond Muffins

Total Time: 45 minutes Serves: 6

1 tsp cinnamon
2 tbsp coconut flour
20 drops liquid stevia
1/4 cup water
1/4 tsp vanilla extract
1/4 tsp baking soda
1/2 tsp baking powder
1/4 cup almond flour
1/2 cup ground flax
2 tbsp ground chia

Preheat the oven to 350 F/ 176 C.
Spray muffin tray with cooking spray and set aside.
In a small bowl, add 6 tablespoons of water and ground chia. Mix well and set aside.
In a mixing bowl, add ground flax, baking soda, baking powder, cinnamon, coconut flour, and almond flour and mix well.
Add chia seed mixture, vanilla, water, and liquid stevia and stir well to combine.

Pour mixture into the prepared muffin tray and bake in preheated oven for 35 minutes.
Serve and enjoy.

Nutritional Value (Amount per Serving): Calories 92; Fat 6.3 g; Carbohydrates 6.9 g; Sugar 0.4 g; Protein 3.7 g; Cholesterol 0 mg

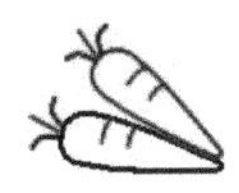

15 Grain-free Overnight Oats

Total Time: 10 minutes Serves: 1

2/3 cup unsweetened coconut milk
2 tsp chia seeds
2 tbsp vanilla protein powder
½ tbsp coconut flour
3 tbsp hemp hearts

Add all ingredients into the glass jar and stir to combine.
Close jar with lid and place in refrigerator for overnight.
Top with fresh berries and serve.

Nutritional Value (Amount per Serving): Calories 378; Fat 22.5 g; Carbohydrates 15 g; Sugar 1.5 g; Protein 27 g; Cholesterol 0 mg

16 Apple Avocado Coconut Smoothie

Total Time: 5 minutes Serves: 2

1 tsp coconut oil
1 tbsp collagen powder
1 tbsp fresh lime juice
½ cup unsweetened coconut milk
¼ apple, slice
1 avocado

Add all ingredients into the blender and blend until smooth and creamy.

Serve and enjoy.

Nutritional Value (Amount per Serving): Calories 262; Fat 23.9 g; Carbohydrates 13.6 g; Sugar 3.4 g; Protein 2 g; Cholesterol 0 mg

17 Chia Cinnamon Smoothie

Total Time: 5 minutes Serves: 1

2 scoops vanilla protein powder
1 tbsp chia seeds
½ tsp cinnamon
1 tbsp coconut oil
½ cup water
½ cup unsweetened coconut milk
Add all ingredients into the blender and blend until smooth and creamy. Serve immediately and enjoy.

Nutritional Value (Amount per Serving): Calories 397; Fat 23.9 g; Carbohydrates 13.4 g; Sugar 0 g; Protein 31.6 g; Cholesterol 0 mg

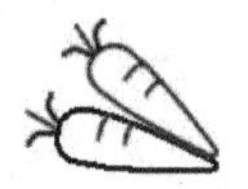

18 Vegetable Tofu Scramble

Total Time: 20 minutes Serves: 2

1 block firm tofu, drained and crumbled
½ tsp turmeric
¼ tsp garlic powder
1 cup spinach
1 red pepper, chopped
10 oz mushrooms, chopped
½ onion, chopped

1 tbsp olive oil
Pepper
Salt

Heat olive oil in a large pan over medium heat.
Add onion, pepper, and mushrooms and sauté until cooked.
Add crumbled tofu, spices, and spinach. Stir well and cook for 3-5 minutes.
Serve and enjoy.

Nutritional Value (Amount per Serving): Calories 159; Fat 9.6 g; Carbohydrates 13.7 g; Sugar 7 g; Protein 9.6 g; Cholesterol 0 mg

19 Strawberry Chia Matcha Pudding

Total Time: 10 minutes Serves: 1

5 drops liquid stevia
2 strawberries, diced
1 ½ tbsp chia seeds
¾ cup unsweetened coconut milk ½
tsp matcha powder

Add all ingredients except strawberries into the glass jar and mix well.
Close jar with lid and place in refrigerator for 4 hours.
Add strawberries into the pudding and mix well.
Serve and enjoy.

Nutritional Value (Amount per Serving): Calories 93; Fat 6.5 g; Carbohydrates 5.6 g; Sugar 1.2 g; Protein 2.5 g; Cholesterol 0 mg

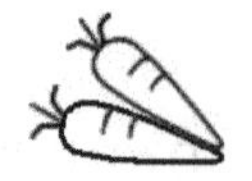

20 Healthy Spinach Green Smoothie

Total Time: 5 minutes Serves: 1

1 cup ice cube
2/3 cup water
½ cup unsweetened almond milk
5 drops liquid stevia
½ tsp matcha powder
1 tsp vanilla extract
1 tbsp MCT oil
½ avocado
2/3 cup spinach

Add all ingredients into the blender and blend until smooth and creamy. Serve immediately and enjoy.

Nutritional Value (Amount per Serving): Calories 167; Fat 18.3 g; Carbohydrates 3.8 g; Sugar 0.6 g; Protein 1.6 g; Cholesterol 0 mg

21 Avocado Chocó Cinnamon Smoothie

Total Time: 5 minutes Serves: 1

½ tsp coconut oil
5 drops liquid stevia
¼ tsp vanilla extract
1 tsp ground cinnamon
2 tsp unsweetened cocoa powder½ avocado

¾ cup unsweetened coconut milk

Add all ingredients into the blender and blend until smooth and creamy. Serve immediately and enjoy.

Nutritional Value (Amount per Serving): Calories 95; Fat 8.3 g; Carbohydrates 5.1 g; Sugar 0.2 g; Protein 1.2 g; Cholesterol 0 mg

22 Protein Breakfast Shake

Total Time: 10 minutes Serves: 2

1 cup coconut milk, unsweetened
1 scoop protein powder
7 oz firm tofu
15 drops liquid stevia
1 tbsp cocoa powder
1 tbsp cocoa nibs
1 tbsp chia seeds
2 tbsp hemp hearts
1/2 oz almonds
Add all ingredients into the blender and blend until you get a thick consistency. Serve and enjoy.

Nutritional Value (Amount per Serving): Calories 243; Fat 13 g; Carbohydrates 11 g; Sugar 1.4 g; Protein 21.2 g; Cholesterol 23 mg

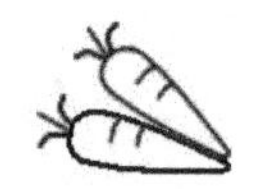

23 Avocado Breakfast Smoothie

Total Time: 5 minutes Serves: 2

5 drops liquid stevia
¼ cup ice cubes
½ avocado
1 tsp vanilla extract
1 cup unsweetened coconut milk

Add all ingredients into the blender and blend until smooth and creamy. Serve immediately and enjoy.

Nutritional Value (Amount per Serving): Calories 131; Fat 11.8 g; Carbohydrates 5.6 g; Sugar 0.5 g; Protein 1 g; Cholesterol 0 mg

24 Almond Coconut Porridge

Total Time: 10 minutes Serves: 2

¾ cup unsweetened almond milk
½ tsp vanilla extract
1 ½ tbsp ground flaxseed
3 tbsp ground almonds
6 tbsp unsweetened shredded coconut Pinch
of sea salt

Add almond milk in microwave safe bowl and microwave for 2 minutes. Add remaining ingredients and stir well and cook for 1 minute. Top with fresh berries and serve.

Nutritional Value (Amount per Serving): Calories 197; Fat 17.4 g; Carbohydrates 8.3 g; Sugar 0.6 g; Protein 4.2 g; Cholesterol 0 mg

25 Cinnamon Muffins

Total Time: 25 minutes Serves: 20

½ cup coconut oil, melted
½ cup pumpkin puree
½ cup almond butter
1 tbsp cinnamon
1 tsp baking powder
2 scoops vanilla protein powder½ cup almond flour

Preheat the oven to 180 C/ 350 F.
Spray muffin tray with cooking spray and set aside.
Add all dry ingredients into the large bowl and mix well.
Add wet ingredients and mix until well combined. Pour batter into the prepared muffin tray and bake in preheated oven for 15 minutes. Serve and enjoy.

Nutritional Value (Amount per Serving): Calories 80; Fat 7.1 g; Carbohydrates 1.6 g; Sugar 0.4 g; Protein 3.5 g; Cholesterol 0 mg

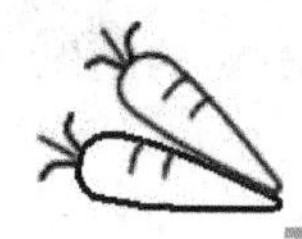

26 Cauliflower Coconut Rice

Total Time: 20 minutes Serves: 3

3 cups cauliflower rice
½ tsp onion powder
1 tsp chili paste
2/3 cup coconut milk
Salt

Add all ingredients to the pan and heat over medium-low heat. Stir to combine.
Cook for 10 minutes. Stir after every 2 minutes.
Remove lid and cook until excess liquid absorbed.
Serve and enjoy.

Nutritional Value (Amount per Serving): Calories 155; Fat 13.1 g; Carbohydrates 9.2 g; Sugar 4.8 g; Protein 3.4 g; Cholesterol 1 mg

27 Fried Okra

Total Time: 20 minutes Serves: 4

1 lb fresh okra, cut into ¼" slices
1/3 cup almond meal
Pepper
Salt
Oil for frying

Heat oil in large pan over medium-high heat.
In a bowl, mix together sliced okra, almond meal, pepper, and salt until well coated.
Once the oil is hot then add okra to the hot oil and cook until lightly browned.
Remove fried okra from pan and allow to drain on paper towels. Serve and enjoy.

Nutritional Value (Amount per Serving): Calories 91; Fat 4.2 g; Carbohydrates 10.2 g; Sugar 10.2 g; Protein 3.9 g; Cholesterol 0 mg

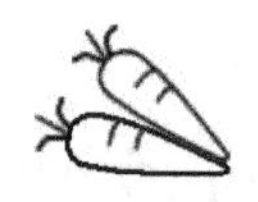

28 Asparagus Mash

Total Time: 20 minutes Serves: 2

10 asparagus shoots, chopped
1 tsp lemon juice
2 tbsp fresh parsley
2 tbsp coconut cream
1 small onion, diced
1 tbsp coconut oil
Pepper
Salt

Sauté onion in coconut oil until onion is softened.
Blanch chopped asparagus in hot water for 2 minutes and drain immediately.
Add sautéed onion, lemon juice, parsley, coconut cream, asparagus, pepper, and salt into the blender and blend until smooth.
Serve warm and enjoy.

Nutritional Value (Amount per Serving): Calories 125; Fat 10.6 g; Carbohydrates 7.5 g; Sugar 3.6 g; Protein 2.6 g; Cholesterol 0 mg

29 Baked Asparagus

Total Time: 25 minutes Serves: 4

40 asparagus spears
2 tbsp vegetable seasoning

2 tbsp garlic powder
2 tbsp salt

Preheat the oven to 450 F/ 232 C.
Arrange all asparagus spears on baking tray and season with vegetable seasoning, garlic powder, and salt.
Place in preheated oven and bake for 20 minutes.
Serve warm and enjoy.

Nutritional Value (Amount per Serving): Calories 75; Fat 0.9 g; Carbohydrates 13.5 g; Sugar 5.5 g; Protein 6.7 g; Cholesterol 0 mg

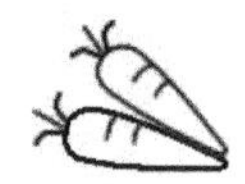

30 Spinach with Coconut Milk

Total Time: 25 minutes Serves: 6

16 oz spinach
2 tsp curry powder
13.5 oz coconut milk
1 tsp lemon zest
½ tsp salt

Add spinach in pan and heat over medium heat. Once it is hot then add curry paste and few tablespoons of coconut milk. Stir well.
Add remaining coconut milk, lemon zest, and salt and cook until thickened.
Serve and enjoy.

Nutritional Value (Amount per Serving): Calories 167; Fat 15.6 g; Carbohydrates 6.7 g; Sugar 2.5 g; Protein 3.7 g; Cholesterol 0 mg

31 Delicious Cabbage Steaks

Total Time: 1 hour 10 minutes Serves: 6

1 medium cabbage head, slice 1" thick
2 tbsp olive oil
1 tbsp garlic, minced
Pepper
Salt
In a small bowl, mix together garlic and olive oil.

Brush garlic and olive oil mixture onto both sides of sliced cabbage.
Season cabbage slices with pepper and salt.
Place cabbage slices onto a baking tray and bake at 350 F/ 180 C for 1 hour.
Turn after 30 minutes.
Serve and enjoy.

Nutritional Value (Amount per Serving): Calories 72; Fat 4.8 g; Carbohydrates 7.4 g; Sugar 3.8 g; Protein 1.6 g; Cholesterol 0 mg

32Garlic Zucchini Squash

Total Time: 20 minutes Serves: 4

1 small squash, sliced
2 tbsp fresh basil, chopped
2 tbsp olive oil
1 garlic clove, chopped
1 large onion, sliced
2 fresh tomatoes, cut into wedges
1 small zucchini, sliced
Pepper
Salt

Heat olive oil in a pan over medium-high heat.
Add onion, squash, zucchini, and garlic and sauté until lightly brown.
Add basil and tomatoes and cook for 5 minutes. Season with pepper and salt.
Simmer over low heat until squash is tender.
Stir well and serve.

Nutritional Value (Amount per Serving): Calories 97; Fat 7.2 g; Carbohydrates 8.2 g; Sugar 4.4 g; Protein 1.4 g; Cholesterol 0 mg

33 Tomato Avocado Cucumber Salad

Total Time: 10 minutes Serves: 4

1 cucumber, sliced
2 avocado, chopped

½ onion, sliced
2 tomatoes,
chopped 1 bell
pepper, chopped For
dressing:
2 tbsp cilantro
¼ tsp garlic powder
2 tbsp olive oil
1 tbsp lemon juice
½ tsp black pepper
½ tsp salt

In a small bowl, mix together all dressing ingredients and set aside.
Add all salad ingredients into the large mixing bowl and mix well.
Pour dressing over salad and toss well.
Serve immediately and enjoy.

Nutritional Value (Amount per Serving): Calories 130; Fat 9.8 g; Carbohydrates 10.6 g; Sugar 5.1 g; Protein 2.1 g; Cholesterol 0 mg

34 Cabbage Coconut Salad

Total Time: 15 minutes Serves: 4

1/3 cup unsweetened desiccated coconut
½ medium head cabbage, shredded
2 tsp sesame seeds
¼ cup tamari sauce
¼ cup olive oil
1 fresh lemon juice

½ tsp cumin
½ tsp curry powder
½ tsp ginger powder

Add all ingredients into the large mixing bowl and toss well.
Place salad bowl in refrigerator for 1 hour.
Serve and enjoy.

Nutritional Value (Amount per Serving): Calories 197; Fat 16.6 g; Carbohydrates 11.4 g; Sugar 7.1 g; Protein 3.5 g; Cholesterol 0 mg

35 Asian Cucumber Salad

Total Time: 10 minutes Serves: 6

4 cups cucumbers, sliced
¼ tsp red pepper flakes
½ tsp sesame oil
1 tsp sesame seeds
¼ cup rice wine vinegar
¼ cup red pepper, diced
¼ cup onion, sliced
½ tsp sea salt

Add all ingredients into the mixing bowl and toss well. Serve immediately and enjoy.

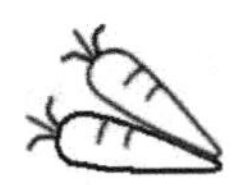

Nutritional Value (Amount per Serving): Calories 27; Fat 0.7 g; Carbohydrates 3.5 g; Sugar 1.6 g; Protein 0.7 g; Cholesterol 0 mg

36 Mexican Cauliflower Rice

Total Time: 25 minutes Serves: 4

1 medium cauliflower head, cut into florets
½ cup tomato sauce
¼ tsp black pepper
1 tsp chili powder
2 garlic cloves, minced
½ medium onion, diced
1 tbsp coconut oil
½ tsp sea salt

Add cauliflower florets into the food processor and process until it looks like rice.

Heat oil in a pan over medium-high heat.
Add onion to the pan and sauté for 5 minutes or until softened.
Add garlic and cook for 1 minute.
Add cauliflower rice, chili powder, pepper, and salt. Stir well.
Add tomato sauce and cook for 5 minutes.
Stir well and serve warm.

Nutritional Value (Amount per Serving): Calories 83; Fat 3.7g; Carbohydrates 11.5 g; Sugar 5.4 g; Protein 3.6 g; Cholesterol 0 mg ;

37 Turnip Salad

Total Time: 10 minutes Serves: 4

4 white turnips, spiralized
1 lemon juice
4 dill sprigs, chopped

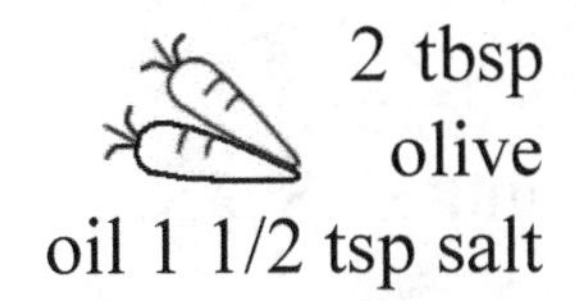 2 tbsp olive oil 1 1/2 tsp salt

Season spiralized turnip with salt and gently massage with hands.
Add lemon juice and dill. Season with pepper and salt.
Drizzle with olive oil and combine everything well.
Serve immediately and enjoy.
Nutritional Value (Amount per Serving): Calories 49; Fat 1.1 g; Carbohydrates 9 g; Sugar 5.2 g; Protein 1.4 g; Cholesterol 0 mg

38 Brussels sprouts Salad

Total Time: 20 minutes Serves: 6

1 ½ lbs Brussels sprouts, trimmed
¼ cup toasted hazelnuts, chopped
2 tsp Dijon mustard
1 ½ tbsp lemon juice
2 tbsp olive oil
Pepper
Salt

In a small bowl, whisk together oil, mustard, lemon juice, pepper, and salt.
In a large bowl, combine together Brussels sprouts and hazelnuts.
Pour dressing over salad and toss well.
Serve immediately and enjoy.

Nutritional Value (Amount per Serving): Calories 111; Fat 7.1 g; Carbohydrates 11 g; Sugar 2.7 g; Protein 4.4 g; Cholesterol 0 mg

39 Tomato Eggplant Spinach Salad

Total Time: 30 minutes Serves: 4

1 large eggplant, cut into 3/4 inch slices
5 oz spinach
1 tbsp sun-dried tomatoes, chopped
1 tbsp oregano, chopped
1 tbsp parsley, chopped
1 tbsp fresh mint, chopped
1 tbsp shallot, chopped
For dressing:

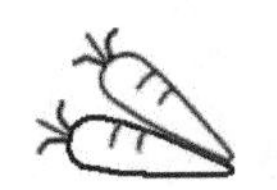

1/4 cup olive oil
1/2 lemon juice
1/2 tsp smoked paprika
1 tsp Dijon mustard
1 tsp tahini
2 garlic cloves, minced
Pepper
Salt

Place sliced eggplants into the large bowl and sprinkle with salt and set aside for minutes.
In a small bowl mix together all dressing ingredients. Set aside.
Heat grill to medium-high heat.
In a large bowl, add shallot, sun-dried tomatoes, herbs, and spinach.
Rinse eggplant slices and pat dry with paper towel.
Brush eggplant slices with olive oil and grill on medium high heat for 3-4 minutes on each side.
Let cool the grilled eggplant slices then cut into quarters.
Add eggplant to the salad bowl and pour dressing over salad. Toss well. Serve and enjoy.

Nutritional Value (Amount per Serving): Calories 163; Fat 13 g; Carbohydrates 10 g; Sugar 3 g; Protein 2 g; Cholesterol 0 mg

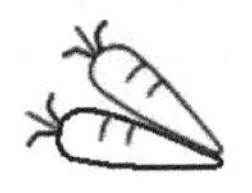

40 Cauliflower Radish Salad

Total Time: 15 minutes Serves: 4

12 radishes, trimmed and chopped
1 tsp dried dill
1 tsp Dijon mustard

1 tbsp cider vinegar
1 tbsp olive oil
1 cup parsley, chopped
½ medium cauliflower head, trimmed and chopped
½ tsp black pepper
¼ tsp sea salt

In a mixing bowl, combine together cauliflower, parsley, and radishes. In a small bowl, whisk together olive oil, dill, mustard, vinegar, pepper, and salt.
Pour dressing over salad and toss well.
Serve immediately and enjoy.

Nutritional Value (Amount per Serving): Calories 58; Fat 3.8 g; Carbohydrates 5.6 g; Sugar 2.1 g; Protein 2.1 g; Cholesterol 0 mg

41 Celery Salad

Total Time: 10 minutes Serves: 6

6 cups celery, sliced
¼ tsp celery seed
1 tbsp lemon juice
2 tsp lemon zest, grated
1 tbsp parsley, chopped
1 tbsp olive oil
Sea salt

Add all ingredients into the large mixing bowl and toss well.
Serve immediately and enjoy.

Nutritional Value (Amount per Serving): Calories 38; Fat 2.5 g; Carbohydrates 3.3 g; Sugar 1.5 g; Protein 0.8 g; Cholesterol 0 mg

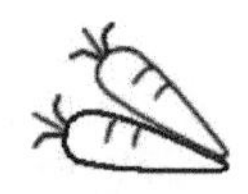

42 Ginger Avocado Kale Salad

Total Time: 15 minutes Serves: 4

1 avocado, peeled and sliced
1 tbsp ginger, grated
1/2 lb kale, chopped
1/4 cup parsley, chopped
2 fresh scallions, chopped

Add all ingredients into the mixing bowl and toss well.
Serve and enjoy.

Nutritional Value (Amount per Serving): Calories 139; Fat 9.9 g; Carbohydrates 12 g; Sugar 0.5 g; Protein 3 g; Cholesterol 0 mg

43 Avocado Cabbage Salad

Total Time: 20 minutes Serves: 4

2 avocados, diced
4 cups cabbage, shredded
3 tbsp fresh parsley, chopped
2 tbsp apple cider vinegar

4 tbsp olive oil
1 cup cherry tomatoes, halved
1/2 tsp pepper
1 1/2 tsp sea salt

Add cabbage, avocados, and tomatoes to a medium bowl and mix well.
In a small bowl, whisk together oil, parsley, vinegar, pepper, and salt.
Pour dressing over vegetables and mix well.
Serve and enjoy.

Nutritional Value (Amount per Serving): Calories 253; Fat 21.6 g; Carbohydrates 14 g; Sugar 4 g; Protein 3.5 g; Cholesterol 0 mg

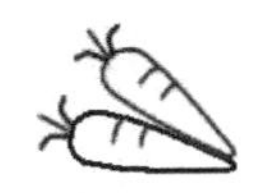

44 Vegetable Salad

Total Time: 15 minutes Serves: 6

2 cups cauliflower florets
2 cups carrots, chopped
2 cups cherry tomatoes, halved
2 tbsp shallots, minced

1 bell pepper, seeded and chopped1 cucumber, seeded and chopped For dressing:
2 garlic cloves, minced
1/2 cup red wine vinegar
1/2 cup olive oil
Pepper
Salt

In a small bowl, combine together all dressing ingredients.
Add all salad ingredients to the large bowl and toss well.
Pour dressing over salad and toss well.
Place salad bowl in refrigerator for 4 hours.
Serve chilled and enjoy.

Nutritional Value (Amount per Serving): Calories 200; Fat 17.1 g; Carbohydrates 12.1 g; Sugar 6.1 g; Protein 2.2 g; Cholesterol 0 mg

45 Refreshing Cucumber Salad

Total Time: 10 minutes Serves: 4

1/3 cup cucumber basil ranch
1 cucumber, chopped
3 tomatoes, chopped
3 tbsp fresh herbs, chopped ½ onion, sliced

Add all ingredients into the large mixing bowl and toss well.
Serve immediately and enjoy.

Nutritional Value (Amount per Serving): Calories 84; Fat 3.4 g;
Carbohydrates 12.5 g; Sugar 6.8 g; Protein 2 g; Cholesterol 0 mg

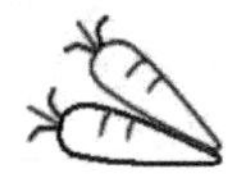

46 Avocado Almond Cabbage Salad

Total Time: 15 minutes Serves: 3

3 cups savoy cabbage, shredded
½ cup blanched almonds
1 avocado, chopped
¼ tsp pepper
¼ tsp sea salt
For dressing:
1 tsp coconut aminos
½ tsp Dijon mustard
1 tbsp lemon juice
3 tbsp olive oil
Pepper
Salt

In a small bowl, mix together all dressing ingredients and set aside.
Add all salad ingredients to the large bowl and mix well.
Pour dressing over salad and toss well.
Serve immediately and enjoy.

Nutritional Value (Amount per Serving): Calories 317; Fat 14.1 g; Carbohydrates 39.8 g; Sugar 9.3 g; Protein 11.6 g; Cholesterol 0 mg

Soups

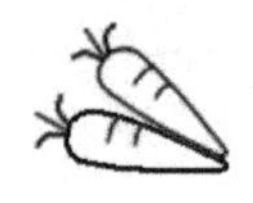

47 Cauliflower Spinach Soup

Total Time: 45 minutes Serves: 5

1/2 cup unsweetened coconut milk
5 oz fresh spinach, chopped
5 watercress, chopped
8 cups vegetable stock
1 lb cauliflower, chopped
Salt

Add stock and cauliflower in a large saucepan and bring to boil over medium heat for 15 minutes.
Add spinach and watercress and cook for another 10 minutes.
Remove from heat and puree the soup using a blender until smooth.
Add coconut milk and stir well. Season with salt.
Stir well and serve hot.

Nutritional Value (Amount per Serving): Calories 153; Fat 8.3 g; Carbohydrates 8.7 g; Sugar 4.3 g; Protein 11.9 g; Cholesterol 0 mg

48 Avocado Mint Soup

Total Time: 10 minutes Serves: 2

1 medium avocado, peeled, pitted, and cut into pieces1 cup coconut milk
2 romaine lettuce leaves
20 fresh mint leaves
1 tbsp fresh lime juice
1/8 tsp salt

Add all ingredients into the blender and blend until smooth. Soup should be thick not as a puree.

Pour into the serving bowls and place in the refrigerator for 10 minutes. Stir well and serve chilled.

Nutritional Value (Amount per Serving): Calories 268; Fat 25.6 g; Carbohydrates 10.2 g; Sugar 0.6 g; Protein 2.7 g; Cholesterol 0 mg

49 Basil Tomato Soup

Total Time: 20 minutes Serves: 6

28 oz can tomatoes
¼ cup basil pesto
¼ tsp dried basil leaves
1 tsp apple cider vinegar
2 tbsp erythritol
¼ tsp garlic powder
½ tsp onion powder
2 cups water
1 ½ tsp kosher salt

Add tomatoes, garlic powder, onion powder, water, and salt in a saucepan.
Bring to boil over medium heat. Reduce heat and simmer for 2 minutes.
Remove saucepan from heat and puree the soup using a blender until smooth.
Stir in pesto, dried basil, vinegar, and erythritol.
Stir well and serve warm.

Nutritional Value (Amount per Serving): Calories 30; Fat 0 g; Carbohydrates 12.1 g; Sugar 9.6 g; Protein 1.3 g; Cholesterol 0 mg

50 Avocado Broccoli Soup

Total Time: 25 minutes Serves: 4

2 cups broccoli florets, chopped
5 cups vegetable broth
2 avocados, chopped
Pepper
Salt

Cook broccoli in boiling water for 5 minutes. Drain well.
Add broccoli, vegetable broth, avocados, pepper, and salt to the blender and blend until smooth. Stir well and serve warm.

Nutritional Value (Amount per Serving): Calories 269; Fat 21.5 g; Carbohydrates 12.8 g; Sugar 2.1 g; Protein 9.2 g; Cholesterol 0 mg

51 Green Spinach Kale Soup

Total Time: 15 minutes Serves: 6

2 avocados
8 oz spinach
8 oz kale
1 fresh lime juice
1 cup water
3 1/3 cup coconut milk
3 oz olive oil
1/4 tsp pepper
1 tsp salt

Heat olive oil in a saucepan over medium heat.
Add kale and spinach to the saucepan and sauté for 2-3 minutes.
Remove saucepan from heat. Add coconut milk, spices, avocado, and water. Stir well.
Puree the soup using an immersion blender until smooth and creamy.
Add fresh lime juice and stir well.
Serve and enjoy.

Nutritional Value (Amount per Serving): Calories 233; Fat 20 g; Carbohydrates 12 g; Sugar 0.5 g; Protein 4.2 g; Cholesterol 0 mg

52 Cauliflower Asparagus Soup

Total Time: 30 minutes Serves: 4

20 asparagus spears, chopped
4 cups vegetable stock
½ cauliflower head, chopped
2 garlic cloves, chopped

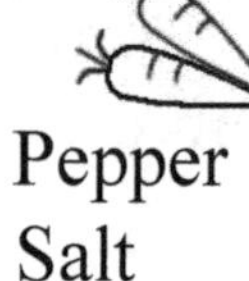

1 tbsp coconut oil

Pepper
Salt

Heat coconut oil in a large saucepan over medium heat.
Add garlic and sauté until softened.
Add cauliflower, vegetable stock, pepper, and salt. Stir well and bring to boil.
Reduce heat to low and simmer for 20 minutes.
Add chopped asparagus and cook until softened.
Puree the soup using an immersion blender until smooth and creamy. Stir well and serve warm.

Nutritional Value (Amount per Serving): Calories 74; Fat 5.6 g; Carbohydrates 8.9 g; Sugar 5.1 g; Protein 3.4 g; Cholesterol 2 mg

53 Creamy Squash Soup

Total Time: 35 minutes Serves: 8

3 cups butternut squash, chopped
1 ½ cups unsweetened coconut milk
1 tbsp coconut oil
1 tsp dried onion flakes
1 tbsp curry powder
4 cups water
1 garlic clove
1 tsp kosher salt

Add squash, coconut oil, onion flakes, curry powder, water, garlic, and salt into a large saucepan. Bring to boil over high heat.
Turn heat to medium and simmer for 20 minutes.
Puree the soup using a blender until smooth. Return soup to the saucepan and stir in coconut milk and cook for 2 minutes.
Stir well and serve hot.

Nutritional Value (Amount per Serving): Calories 146; Fat 12.6 g; Carbohydrates 9.4 g; Sugar 2.8 g; Protein 1.7 g; Cholesterol 0 mg

54Zucchini Soup

Total Time: 20 minutes Serves: 8

2 ½ lbs zucchini, peeled and sliced
1/3 cup basil leaves
4 cups vegetable stock
4 garlic cloves, chopped

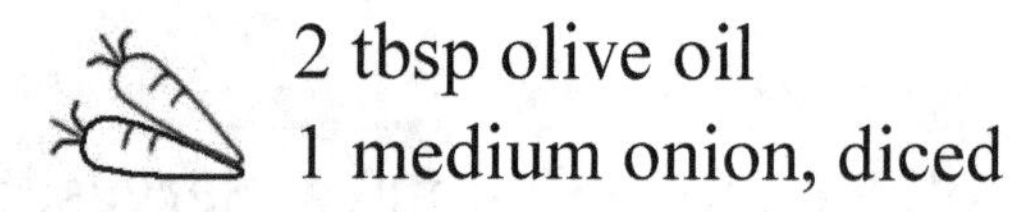
2 tbsp olive oil
1 medium onion, diced

Pepper
Salt

Heat olive oil in a pan over medium-low heat.
Add zucchini and onion and sauté until softened. Add garlic and sauté for a minute.
Add vegetable stock and simmer for 15 minutes.
Remove from heat. Stir in basil and puree the soup using a blender until smooth and creamy. Season with pepper and salt.
Stir well and serve.

Nutritional Value (Amount per Serving): Calories 62; Fat 4 g; Carbohydrates 6.8 g; Sugar 3.3 g; Protein 2 g; Cholesterol 0 mg

55 Creamy Celery Soup

Total Time: 40 minutes Serves: 4

6 cups celery
½ tsp dill
2 cups water
1 cup coconut milk
1 onion, chopped
Pinch of salt

Add all ingredients into the instant pot and stir well.
Cover instant pot with lid and select soup setting.
Release pressure using quick release method than open the lid.

Puree the soup using an immersion blender until smooth and creamy. Stir well and serve warm.

Nutritional Value (Amount per Serving): Calories 174; Fat 14.6 g; Carbohydrates 10.5 g; Sugar 5.2 g; Protein 2.8 g; Cholesterol 0 mg

56 Tomato Pumpkin Soup

Total Time: 25 minutes Serves: 4

2 cups pumpkin, diced
1/2 cup tomato, chopped
1/2 cup onion, chopped
1 1/2 tsp curry powder1/2 tsp paprika
2 cups vegetable stock
1 tsp olive oil
1/2 tsp garlic, minced

In a saucepan, add oil, garlic, and onion and sauté for 3 minutes over medium heat.
Add remaining ingredients into the saucepan and bring to boil.
Reduce heat and cover and simmer for 10 minutes.
Puree the soup using a blender until smooth.
Stir well and serve warm.
Nutritional Value (Amount per Serving): Calories 70; Fat 2.7 g; Carbohydrates 13.8 g; Sugar 6.3 g; Protein 1.9 g; Cholesterol 0 mg

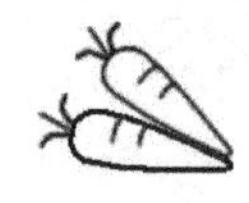

57 Avocado Cucumber Soup

Total Time: 40 minutes Serves: 3

1 large cucumber, peeled and sliced
¾ cup water
¼ cup lemon juice
2 garlic cloves
6 green onion
2 avocados, pitted
½ tsp black pepper
½ tsp pink salt

Add all ingredients into the blender and blend until smooth and creamy.
Place in refrigerator for 30 minutes.
Stir well and serve chilled.

Nutritional Value (Amount per Serving): Calories 73; Fat 3.7 g; Carbohydrates 9.2 g; Sugar 2.8 g; Protein 2.2 g; Cholesterol 0 mg

58 Creamy Garlic Onion Soup

Total Time: 45 minutes Serves: 4

1 onion, sliced
4 cups vegetable stock
1 1/2 tbsp olive oil
1 shallot, sliced
2 garlic clove, chopped
1 leek, sliced
Salt

Add stock and olive oil in a saucepan and bring to boil.
Add remaining ingredients and stir well.
Cover and simmer for 25 minutes.
Puree the soup using an immersion blender until smooth.
Stir well and serve warm.

Nutritional Value (Amount per Serving): Calories 90; Fat 7.4 g; Carbohydrates 10.1 g; Sugar 4.1 g; Protein 1 g; Cholesterol 0 mg

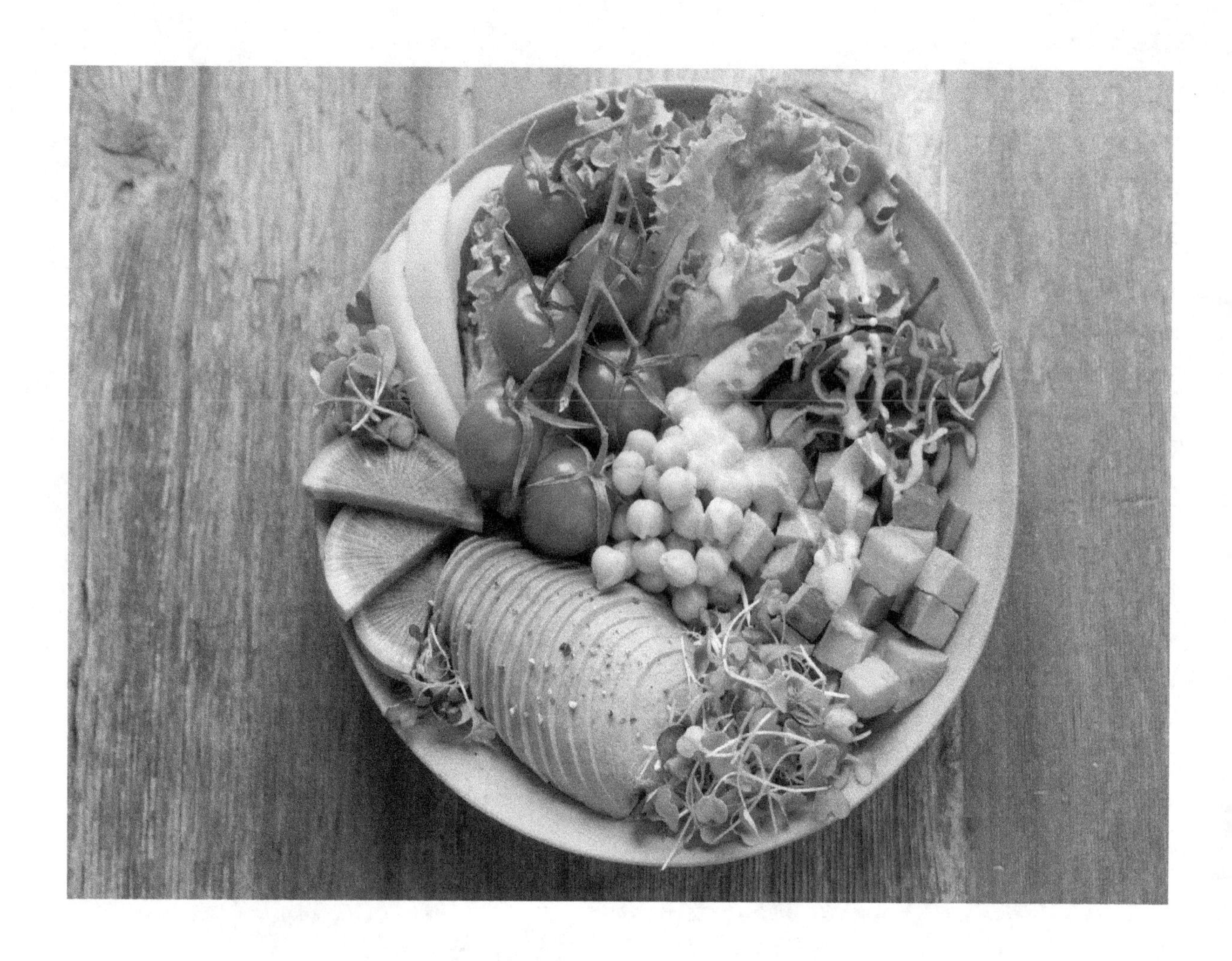

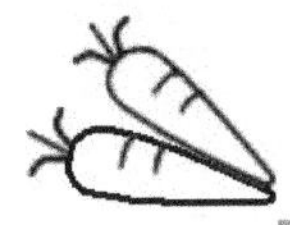

59 Avocado Pudding

Total Time: 10 minutes Serves: 8

2 ripe avocados, peeled, pitted and cut into pieces
1 tbsp fresh lime juice
14 oz can coconut milk
80 drops of liquid stevia
2 tsp vanilla extract

Add all ingredients into the blender and blend until smooth.
Serve and enjoy.

Nutritional Value (Amount per Serving): Calories 317; Fat 30.1 g; Carbohydrates 9.3 g; Sugar 0.4 g; Protein 3.4 g; Cholesterol 0 mg

60 Almond Butter Brownies

Total Time: 30 minutes Serves: 4

1 scoop protein powder
2 tbsp cocoa powder
1/2 cup almond butter, melted
1 cup bananas, overripe

Preheat the oven to 350 F/ 176 C.
Spray brownie tray with cooking spray.

Add all ingredients into the blender and blend until smooth. Pour batter into the prepared dish and bake in preheated oven for 20 minutes. Serve and enjoy.

Nutritional Value (Amount per Serving): Calories 82; Fat 2.1 g; Carbohydrates 11.4 g; Protein 6.9 g; Sugars 5 g; Cholesterol 16 mg

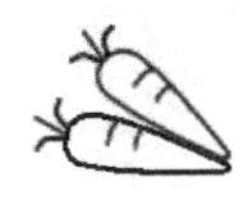

61 Raspberry Chia Pudding

Total Time: 3 hours 10 minutes Serves: 2

4 tbsp chia seeds
1 cup coconut milk
1/2 cup raspberries

Add raspberry and coconut milk in a blender and blend until smooth.
Pour mixture into the Mason jar.
Add chia seeds in a jar and stir well.
Close jar tightly with lid and shake well.
Place in refrigerator for 3 hours.
Serve chilled and enjoy.

Nutritional Value (Amount per Serving): Calories 361; Fat 33.4 g; Carbohydrates 13.3 g; Sugar 5.4 g; Protein 6.2 g; Cholesterol 0 mg

62 Chocolate Fudge

Total Time: 10 minutes Serves: 12

4 oz unsweetened dark chocolate
3/4 cup coconut butter
15 drops liquid stevia
1 tsp vanilla extract

Melt coconut butter and dark chocolate.
Add ingredients to the large bowl and combine well.
Pour mixture into a silicone loaf pan and place in refrigerator until set. Cut into pieces and serve.

Nutritional Value (Amount per Serving): Calories 157; Fat 14.1 g; Carbohydrates 6.1 g; Sugar 1 g; Protein 2.3 g; Cholesterol 0 mg

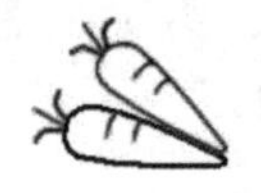

63 Quick Chocó Brownie

Total Time: 10 minutes Serves: 1

1/4 cup almond milk
1 tbsp cocoa powder
1 scoop chocolate protein powder
1/2 tsp baking powder

In a microwave-safe mug blend together baking powder, protein powder, and cocoa.
Add almond milk in a mug and stir well.
Place mug in microwave and microwave for 30 seconds.
Serve and enjoy.

Nutritional Value (Amount per Serving): Calories 207; Fat 15.8 g; Carbohydrates 9.5 g; Sugar 3.1 g; Protein 12.4 g; Cholesterol 20 mg

64 Simple Almond Butter Fudge

Total Time: 15 minutes Serves: 8

1/2 cup almond butter

15 drops liquid stevia
2 1/2 tbsp coconut oil

Combine together almond butter and coconut oil in a saucepan. Gently warm until melted.
Add stevia and stir well.
Pour mixture into the candy container and place in refrigerator until set. Serve and enjoy.

Nutritional Value (Amount per Serving): Calories 43; Fat 4.8 g; Carbohydrates 0.2 g; Protein 0.2 g; Sugars 0 g; Cholesterol 0 mg

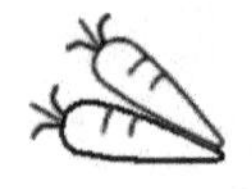

65 Coconut Peanut Butter Fudge

Total Time: 1 hour 15 minutes Serves: 20

12 oz smooth peanut butter
3 tbsp coconut oil
4 tbsp coconut cream
15 drops liquid stevia
Pinch of salt

Line baking tray with parchment paper.
Melt coconut oil in a saucepan over low heat.
Add peanut butter, coconut cream, stevia, and salt in a saucepan. Stir well.
Pour fudge mixture into the prepared baking tray and place in refrigerator for 1 hour.
Cut into pieces and serve.

Nutritional Value (Amount per Serving): Calories 125; Fat 11.3 g; Carbohydrates 3.5 g; Sugar 1.7 g; Protein 4.3 g; Cholesterol 0 mg

66 Lemon Mousse

Total Time: 10 minutes Serves: 2

14 oz coconut milk
12 drops liquid stevia
1/2 tsp lemon extract
1/4 tsp turmeric

Place coconut milk can in the refrigerator for overnight. Scoop out thick cream into a mixing bowl.
Add remaining ingredients to the bowl and whip using a hand mixer until smooth.
Transfer mousse mixture to a zip-lock bag and pipe into small serving glasses. Place in refrigerator.
Serve chilled and enjoy.

Nutritional Value (Amount per Serving): Calories 444; Fat 45.7 g; Carbohydrates 10 g; Sugar 6 g; Protein 4.4 g; Cholesterol 0 mg

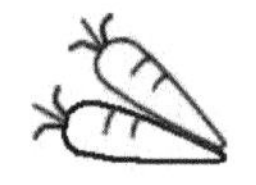

67 Chocó Chia Pudding

Total Time: 10 minutes Serves: 6

2 1/2 cups coconut milk
2 scoops stevia extract powder
6 tbsp cocoa powder
1/2 cup chia seeds
1/2 tsp vanilla extract
1/8 cup xylitol
1/8 tsp salt

Add all ingredients into the blender and blend until smooth.

Pour mixture into the glass container and place in refrigerator. Serve chilled and enjoy.

Nutritional Value (Amount per Serving): Calories 259; Fat 25.4 g; Carbohydrates 10.2 g; Sugar 3.5 g; Protein 3.8 g; Cholesterol 0 mg

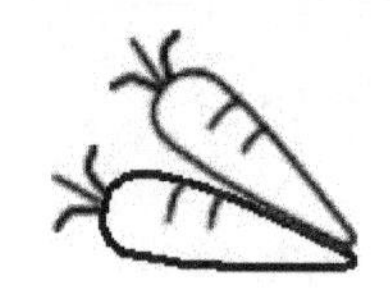

68 Almond Green Beans

Total Time: 20 minutes Serves: 4

1 lb fresh green beans, trimmed
1/3 cup almonds, sliced
4 garlic cloves, sliced
2 tbsp olive oil
1 tbsp lemon juice
½ tsp sea salt

Add green beans, salt, and lemon juice in a mixing bowl. Toss well and set aside.
Heat oil in a pan over medium heat.
Add sliced almonds and sauté until lightly browned.
Add garlic and sauté for 30 seconds.
Pour almond mixture over green beans and toss well.
Stir well and serve immediately.

Nutritional Value (Amount per Serving): Calories 146; Fat 11.2 g; Carbohydrates 10.9 g; Sugar 2 g; Protein 4 g; Cholesterol 0 mg

69 Cinnamon Oatmeal

Total Time: 10 minutes Serves: 2

¾ cup hot water
2 tbsp. sugar-free maple syrup
½ tsp. ground cinnamon
2 tbsp. ground flax seeds
3 tbsp. vegan vanilla protein powder3 tbsp hulled hemp seeds

Add all ingredients into the bowl and stir until well combined. Serve and enjoy.

Nutritional Value (Amount per Serving): Calories 220; Fat 12.5 g; Carbohydrates 9.5 g; Sugar 0.1 g; Protein 17.6 g; Cholesterol 0 mg

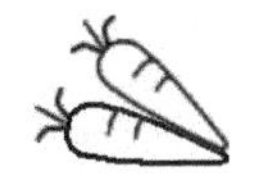

70 Zucchini Muffins

Total Time: 35 minutes Serves: 8

1 cup almond flour
1 zucchini, grated
1/4 cup coconut oil, melted
15 drops liquid stevia
1/2 tsp baking soda

1/2 cup coconut flour
1/2 cup walnut, chopped
1 1/2 tsp cinnamon
3/4 cup unsweetened applesauce
1/8 tsp salt

Preheat the oven to 325 F/ 162 C.
Spray muffin tray with cooking spray and set aside.
In a bowl, combine together grated zucchini, coconut oil, and stevia. In another bowl, mix together coconut flour, baking soda, almond flour, walnut, cinnamon, and salt.
Add zucchini mixture into the coconut flour mixture and mix well.
Add applesauce and stir until well combined.
Pour batter into the prepared muffin tray and bake in preheated oven for 2530 minutes.
Serve and enjoy.

Nutritional Value (Amount per Serving): Calories 229; Fat 18.9 g; Carbohydrates 12.5 g; Sugar 3.4 g; Protein 5.2 g; Cholesterol 0 mg

71 Healthy Breakfast Granola

Total Time: 15 minutes Serves: 5

1 cup walnuts, diced
1 cup unsweetened coconut flakes
1 cup sliced almonds
2 tbsp coconut oil, melted
4 packets Splenda
2 tsp cinnamon

Preheat the oven to 375 F/ 190 C.
Spray a baking tray with cooking spray and set aside.
Add all ingredients into the medium bowl and toss well.
Spread bowl mixture on a prepared baking tray and bake in preheated oven for 10 minutes. Serve and enjoy.

Nutritional Value (Amount per Serving): Calories 458; Fat 42.5 g; Carbohydrates 13.7 g; Sugar 2.7 g; Protein 11.7 g; Cholesterol 0 mg

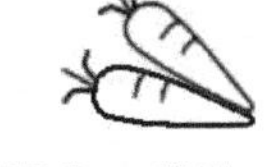

72 Chia Flaxseed Waffles

Total Time: 25 minutes Serves: 8

2 cups ground golden flaxseed
2 tsp cinnamon
10 tsp ground chia seed
15 tbsp warm water
1/3 cup coconut oil, melted
1/2 cup water
1 tbsp baking powder
1 tsp sea salt

Preheat the waffle iron.
In a small bowl, mix together ground chia seed and warm water.
In a large bowl, mix together ground flax seed, sea salt, and baking powder. Set aside.

Add melted coconut oil, chia seed mixture, and water into the blender and blend for 30 seconds.
Transfer coconut oil mixture into the flax seed mixture and mix well. Add cinnamon and stir well.
Scoop waffle mixture into the hot waffle iron and cook on each side for 3-5 minutes. Serve and enjoy.

Nutritional Value (Amount per Serving): Calories 240; Fat 20.6 g; Carbohydrates 12.9 g; Sugar 0 g; Protein 7 g; Cholesterol 0 mg

73 Baked Cauliflower

Total Time: 55 minutes Serves: 2

1/2 cauliflower head, cut into florets
2 tbsp olive oil For seasoning:
1/2 tsp garlic powder
1/2 tsp ground cumin
1/2 tsp black pepper
1/2 tsp white pepper
1 tsp onion powder
1/4 tsp dried oregano
1/4 tsp dried basil
1/4 tsp dried thyme
1 tbsp ground cayenne pepper
2 tbsp ground paprika2 tsp salt
Preheat the oven to 400 F/ 200 C.
Spray a baking tray with cooking spray and set aside.
In a large bowl, mix together all seasoning ingredients.
Add oil and stir well. Add cauliflower to the bowl seasoning mixture and stir well to coat.
Spread the cauliflower florets on a baking tray and bake in preheated oven for 45 minutes. Serve and enjoy.

Nutritional Value (Amount per Serving): Calories 177; Fat 15.6 g; Carbohydrates 11.5 g; Sugar 3.2 g; Protein 3.1 g; Cholesterol 0 mg

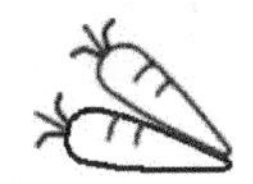

74 Sage Pecan Cauliflower

Total Time: 40 minutes Serves: 6

1 large cauliflower head, cut into florets
1/2 tsp dried thyme
1/2 tsp poultry seasoning
1/4 cup olive oil
2 garlic clove, minced
1/4 cup pecans, chopped
2 tbsp parsley, chopped
1/2 tsp ground sage
1/4 cup celery, chopped
1 onion, sliced
1/4 tsp black pepper
1 tsp sea salt

Preheat the oven to 450 F/ 232 C.
Spray a baking tray with cooking spray and set aside.
In a large bowl, mix together cauliflower, thyme, poultry seasoning, olive oil, garlic, celery, sage, onions, pepper, and salt.
Spread mixture on a baking tray and roast in preheated oven for 15 minutes.
Add pecans and parsley and stir well. Roast for 10-15 minutes more. Serve and enjoy.

Nutritional Value (Amount per Serving): Calories 118; Fat 8.6 g; Carbohydrates 9.9 g; Sugar 4.2 g; Protein 3.1 g; Cholesterol 0 mg

75 Herb Spaghetti Squash

Total Time: minutes Serves: 4

4 cups spaghetti squash, cooked
½ tsp pepper
½ tsp sage
1 tsp dried parsley
1 tsp dried thyme
1 tsp dried rosemary
1 tsp garlic powder
2 tbsp olive oil
1 tsp salt

Preheat the oven to 350 F/ 180 C.
Add all ingredients into the mixing bowl and mix well to combine.
Transfer bowl mixture to the oven safe dish and cook in preheated oven for 15 minutes.
Stir well and serve.

Nutritional Value (Amount per Serving): Calories 96; Fat 7.7 g; Carbohydrates 8.1 g; Sugar 0.2 g; Protein 0.9 g; Cholesterol 0 mg

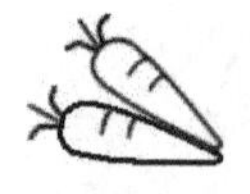

76 Cauliflower Couscous

Total Time: 25 minutes Serves: 4

1 head cauliflower, cut into florets
14 black olives
1 garlic cloves, chopped
14 oz can artichokes
2 tbsp olive oil
1/4 cup parsley, chopped
1 lemon juice
1/2 tsp pepper
1/2 tsp salt

Preheat the oven to 400 F/ 200 C.
Add cauliflower florets into the food processor and process until it looks like rice.
Spread cauliflower rice on a baking tray and drizzle with olive oil. Bake in preheated oven for 12 minutes.
In a bowl, mix together garlic, lemon juice, artichokes, parsley, and olives.
Add cauliflower to the bowl and stir well. Season with pepper and salt. Serve and enjoy.

Nutritional Value (Amount per Serving): Calories 116; Fat 8.8 g; Carbohydrates 8.4 g; Sugar 3.3 g; Protein 3.3 g; Cholesterol 0 mg

77 Classic Cabbage Slaw

Total Time: 20 minutes Serves: 3

4 cups green cabbage, shredded
2 garlic cloves
1 tbsp sesame oil
2 tbsp tamari
1 tsp vinegar
1 tsp chili paste
½ cup macadamia nuts, chopped

Toss shredded green cabbage in a pan with chili paste, sesame oil, vinegar, and tamari on medium-low heat.
Add garlic and cook for 5 minutes or until cabbage is softened.
Stir everything well. Add macadamia nuts and cook for 5 minutes. Stir well and serve.

Nutritional Value (Amount per Serving): Calories 240; Fat 21.8 g; Carbohydrates 10.5 g; Sugar 4.7 g; Protein 4.5 g; Cholesterol 1 mg

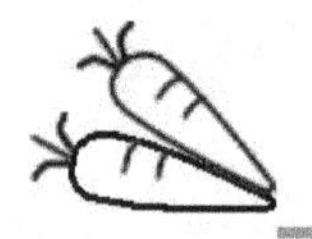

78 Lemon Garlic Mushrooms

Total Time: 25 minutes Serves: 4

3 oz enoki mushrooms
1 tbsp olive oil
1 tsp lemon zest, chopped
2 tbsp lemon juice
3 garlic cloves, sliced
6 oyster mushrooms, halved
5 oz cremini mushrooms, sliced
1/2 red chili, sliced

1/2 onion, sliced
1 tsp sea salt

Heat olive oil in a pan over high heat.
Add shallots, enoki mushrooms, oyster mushrooms, cremini mushrooms, and chili.
Stir well and cook over medium-high heat for 10 minutes.
Add lemon zest and stir well. Season with lemon juice and salt and cook for 3-4 minutes.
Serve and enjoy.

Nutritional Value (Amount per Serving): Calories 87; Fat 5.6 g; Carbohydrates 7.5 g; Sugar 1.8 g; Protein 3 g; Cholesterol 8 mg

Chapter 5 How to use the included meal plan

Prepping your meals is a real game changer. As in many of life's pursuits, forming habits will yield the best results, so develop a routine right from the start. Pick one or two days per week when you can dedicate 2-4 hours to cooking. (Choose two days rather than one if you have limited storage space or smaller time windows per day.) Make sure to have all ingredients ready and prepare labels for each meal you're about to prep.

Keep a Schedule

Keeping a schedule in your agenda, notebook, or smartphone will help you remember what to eat at your predetermined dates and times. Label all prepped dishes according to this schedule. Write both the recipe name and the date you plan to eat it on the label and on your schedule. This will reduce confusion, and you can avoid consulting your meal plan each time you sit down to eat. Proper labeling and writing down your meals for the day will make it super easy to stick to your plan, reduce stress, and reach your fitness goals!

Following the meal plan strictly, for the full 30 days, can require you to prepare up to 25 recipes per week. But this is not necessary; the best way to follow the meal plan in this book is to pick one or two days with recipes you enjoy and prep these recipes for multiple days in row.

Macronutrients and daily calorie intake

Each day of the meal plan guarantees a proper number of balanced macronutrients. Depending on your nutritional needs, you can determine the appropriate number of servings. Choose two or more daily sets of recipes that you can alternate throughout the week, so you can have variety while only needing to prepare four to eight recipes per prepping session.

Following a meal plan doesn't have to be boring; you can change your preferences each week.

Each day in the included meal plan consists of five meals: breakfast, two snacks, lunch, and dinner. These meals may vary in serving size. The daily meal plan provides portions for 1600, 1800, 2000, 2500 or 3000 kcal per day. Depending on your bodyweight and goals, it's important to aim for a calorie deficit for weight loss, or a surplus of calories and macros for muscle growth. Consuming one gram of protein per day for each lean pound of your body weight is recommended for gaining muscle. If your meals on a given day of the meal plan don't deliver enough protein, you can supplement with one or more protein shakes. Note that these shakes also have nutritional value, so this calorie amount should be included in the total daily calories. Always keep track of your macronutrient and calorie intake and physical results, but keep in mind that small changes won't affect your weight or progress right away.

If you want to make any changes to the meal plan, which is not recommended, it's important to stick to the given macro balances. If you want to replace one or more meals because you don't like them, recalculate the macro values and swap in equivalent meals from different days of the plan. A notepad will make it easy to recalculate macro values.

Tip: Use an app, Excel sheet, or a notepad to keep track of your macro intake. This will save you headaches and guarantee the right number of macros for every day of the week. Some great apps include MyMacros+, MyFitnessPal and Nutritionist.

Ultimately, the goal is to find a meal prepping routine that works for you. Cook on days that you prefer, but always plan ahead of time to prevent an empty fridge or freezer. You have the flexibility to interchange days of the meal plan but stick to the prescribed portion sizes and macro amounts, and keep track of your macronutrient and calorie intake.

Make meal prepping a habitual part of your lifestyle and you'll find it a lot easier to reach your health and fitness goals!

Creating a matching shopping list and grocery shopping

Create a shopping list to optimize each trip to the grocery store. First, make sure to list all the ingredients required for the recipes you plan to prepare in your upcoming prepping session(s). Remember that you can choose to prep either once or twice per week. You can buy all the ingredients for the entire week in a single grocery shopping session but do consider the expiration date of ingredients. You might want to buy fresh ingredients with a limited shelf life more often than once a week.

Another thing to consider is your pantry. A seasoned meal prepper keeps his or her pantry stocked with nonperishables and keeps track of what is running low or nearing expiration.

Make sure that on each trip to the grocery store (or stores, if you buy your ingredients in different places), you bring a list and stick to it. Preparing a complete list will ensure that you have all the ingredients required when it's time to cook the dishes on prepping days. Buying only what's necessary will help you save money and prevent waste.

Save your lists to a cloud storage service like Google Drive so you can access them anytime and anywhere with your smartphone. This way, you'll always be able to access it during your shopping trip. Alternatively, you can sign up for a grocery delivery service like Amazon Prime or Instacart. These apps enable you to save your list in the app and have all your groceries delivered before you start cooking for the next week of meal prep!

Chapter 6 Prepping and Storing Food

The freezer is one of the most useful devices when meal prepping but to make life easier, there are some things to keep in mind. It is a good idea to regularly clean out your freezer. Store your food at room temperature or in the refrigerator before freezing so that your food is not hot when you put it in-which thaws the ice and food around it.

Keeping the freezer full is more economical and air will be kept cold more easily but don't overload it so that no air can circulate. Be careful not to keep the door open for long when taking food in and out as the food inside will start to defrost and go bad.

Vegan ingredients that are easy to prepare

Vegetables and Beans

Blanch your beans and vegetables before freezing them to preserve their color, texture and flavor. Cooked vegetable purees and beans can also go into the freezer. The blanching process is explained below.

Fruit

Frozen fruits are great for smoothies. Fruits that freeze well include apples, olives, avocados, pears, kiwis, oranges, grapefruit, lemons, limes, peaches, plums, nectarines, bananas, raspberries, blackberries, watermelon, honeydew melons, cantaloupe, apricots, grapes, mangoes, cherries, strawberries, blueberries, raisins, currants, cranberries, dates and figs.

Other vegan foods that can be frozen

Seeds that can be frozen include: almonds, cashews, walnuts, pecans, sunflower seeds, sunflower seed butter, pumpkin seeds, chia seeds, ground flaxseed and sesame seeds.

Herbs and spices such as oregano, thyme, cumin, turmeric, chili powder, cinnamon, pepper, salsa, soy sauce and mustard are also freezer-friendly. To freeze herbs, remove the leaves from the stems and allow the herbs to dry by leaving them out in the air. After drying, place the herbs in a bag and into the freezer.

Grains, beans and legumes also freeze well. Vegetables like peas, runner, French, dwarf and broad beans, asparagus and broccoli can go into the freezer as well.

What not to freeze

Vegetables high in water content, including cucumber, lettuce, bean sprouts, cauliflower florets, zucchini and tomatoes do not freeze well and must be blanched first. If they are not blanched, they become limp or mushy when thawed. Herbs like basil, chives and parsley will suffer from freezer burn. Carrots will become rubbery if frozen and potatoes, unless they are cooked first, will undergo texture change.

What is Blanching?

Blanching involves rapid heating and cooling to remove moisture from a vegetable. Vegetables are placed in a blanching pot basket surrounded by boiling water. After 2 minutes, the basket is removed and quickly transferred to a tub of cold water before being drained. Vegetables are then ready to put in the freezer.

Chapter 7 Tips for Staying on Track

One thing that I have heard so many people worry and stress about when beginning to adopt a vegan diet is that they will miss the meat, or they're worried about how to get the protein and iron. I've even had so many friends think they couldn't do it because they would miss meat so much and they were scared they wouldn't be able to keep it up over time. So whether you're just becoming a vegan now or you already are one, we're going to tell you how to start on this diet and how to stay on this diet. The one thing I recommend the most is if you're really worried about cutting meat from your diet, go slow. Also, if it helps, there are so many yummy alternatives to meat and you can find them at just about any supermarket which should make the switch even easier. Another thing to remind people is that once you begin adjusting to this diet, you will probably begin to crave meat less and less. Many people have said that they have been vegan for most of their lives and don't miss meat at all. Others say they feel bad for the meat eaters who are missing out on what vegetarians and vegans enjoy every day, from the great health benefits of the food to the wonderful flavors of the new foods in their diet.

A good tip to start out is do not go cold turkey. No pun intended. When you go cold turkey without adequate preparation, you tend to be more likely to go back to eating meat and your old diet. Then you feel guilty and it can be a bad cycle. Removing it slowly over time is the best way to go about this because you're familiarizing your body to the new food and letting go of the old. Over time, you'll notice that you're craving meat less and the switch will become easier. A good example to go with is let's say you're trying to cut sweets out of your diet. So you remove anything with sugar in your house. Then you start to eat healthy for maybe a few hours or a day and you begin to get cravings. The problem with many people is that they get so hungry because they don't have the proper research about what to eat, and then they end up going on a binge or running out to the nearest place with cookies or they stay home, and binge eat. Now, you might think binging on healthy food is better but it's not. Binge eating is never healthy and can lead to eating disorders which are a bad thing.

Later, you feel guilty and ashamed which only hurts you and your progress as well as your emotional being. If you slip up, remember you are human. It can happen to anyone and there is no reason to feel guilty or ashamed. Slipups happen. The best thing we can do is to try again on the diet and try your best not to slip up. It is also important to note that slip-ups will probably happen in the first couple of days and if they do, it's alright. The important thing is that you're trying to better yourself and that you want to change. This is a good thing. Reminding yourself of that will help guide you because you will be able to understand that the effort you're putting forth is something to be proud of and one day you won't slip up at all.

You should also begin adding to your diet before taking things away. Familiarize yourself with how you prepare your new food, how it's stored, and the uses they have. With studying, you will see that many of your items can be used as multipurpose items. Olive oil is great for your skin and hair just as one example of how it can be used in a different way. You should start adding more vegan staples but keep in mind that you're a vegan and ketogenic, not just one or the other. This means that there are certain things that ketogenic eat that vegans don't; like fish or meat for ketogenic; for vegans, most eat beans or potatoes and starchy foods but ketogenic usually avoid them because of the high carb content. So when adding things to your

diet, keep in mind what you need to avoid and what will bring the most benefits to your new lifestyle.
A fun way to get yourself used to this new lifestyle is to experiment with different recipes that sound good to you. You'll either realize that you like it and want to eat it again or maybe share it with the people around you if you live with others. Or maybe, instead, you'll be able to tell that it's something you don't like and wouldn't want to try again. Or maybe, it's just something you didn't like cooking. In that case, if you liked the dish but didn't like the work it took to prepare it, which happens to many people, that might lead you to a new restaurant that has the foods you can eat, and you might like how they prepare it. Once you begin experimenting and getting comfortable making the meals, it will become easier to adopt a new diet and find new foods that you like.

You can alter the recipes you already have and use on a daily basis too. If you eat meals with meat, make them vegetarian and then make them vegan before final making them ketogenic or Keto for short. You're still eating a meal that you already enjoy; it is just a different version of it. This can help you with your transition because it's just adapting things you're already used to. An example would be chili. Chili doesn't have to include meat at all, but if you really want it, try a meat substitute. Since beans aren't good for ketogenic because most of them are high in carbs, be sure to go through those carefully looking into the carb content and find a better option for that part of the diet as well. You could come up with an amazing recipe no one ever thought of before or you might be willing to try recipes that you wouldn't before this.

As you adapt to this lifestyle more and more, you should be able to stay on it much easier. Some good tips for maintaining your vegan lifestyle is if you

like to eat out, it's like we said it can be difficult with your eating needs. So find out in advance where you can and can't go.
Have special food you can take with you when you leave your house. More and more places are trying to accommodate people's needs but some just don't have everything that you are able to eat because your diet can be a little bit restrictive. This is really going to help you keep yourself from being tempted by other's influence or choices or if a place you're at can't meet the needs of your diet. When you're out at social situations, it can be tempting to get out of your diet or eat foods you know you shouldn't. We have all been there. You can be at a dinner with a few friends and they want to share an appetizer and you think one won't hurt, or they want to drink so you figure one drink won't have too many carbs or something along those lines. A quick tip though; a lot of drinks do have carbs and on a ketogenic diet, it is really not recommended because you'll bust straight through your numbers. Some people even give in to the peer pressure because their friends get upset that someone is not eating like the rest of them. Ignore the peer pressure and do what you want to do. You don't have to answer to anyone but yourself.

Getting support will help you be able to stick to your diet as well. Having people around that love you and support you can be a very big help during this transition. Family can be a big help when you're making such a drastic change. If you are not able to be around encouraging people, then be sure to find motivation and encourage yourself. Too many diets come with negativity and people making fun of others for trying something different. If this is what happens to you, I am sorry because no one deserves that at all and it can be very painful for someone to have to go through. The best thing you can do is ignore the hate and keep a positive attitude and remember what you're doing this for. You're doing this for you, not them, and you don't need their negativity. Ignore it and brush it off and stick to what you really want.

I know it can be difficult but just remember you don't need to keep that negativity around you and you are stronger than they are. You are the one that lives your life and you should be happy. Remember this and just keep pushing through. I recommend a reward for you as well. For instance, if you managed to stay a vegan ketogenic for a month, reward yourself with something you've been wanting, like a new pair of shoes or a movie that you've wanted to see. The act of giving yourself a reward will send a positive vibe to your brain that will reinforce your healthy habits and help you to want to keep going on your journey.

Make sure you stay informed. You need to make sure you've got good information going into this because that will help you know what you can and can't eat, or wear or use on your body. Also, stay up to date on science and studies. People are still researching these diets and lifestyles to give people the correct information. If you stay up to date, you'll be able to see the new information too.

If you feel like you can't do it, remind yourself why you decided to do this in the first place. Remind yourself of the facts. Watch videos online or read studies. They say it's harder to slip when you see the facts presented to you and you're watching the consequences of eating meat.

Offer to make dinner for your friends or ask if you can make some vegan dishes to a dinner or party. More often than not, you will see that they're really interested in what you have to say and that they will love how amazing your food tastes. They may even opt to go vegan themselves! A perfect example is let's say all your meat-eater friends are having a dinner party and wants you to bring a dessert. Okay, easy peasy. Make them some vegan keto zucchini brownies, or some vegan keto cupcakes and watch them fall in love.

I bet you won't even be able to tell that there are healthy vegetables in there and your friends will fall in love.
Make your lifestyle the new norm. Everyone thinks that meat-eating is the norm; switch what it means. Now, this doesn't mean getting in people's faces and being rude or abrupt. Be kind and polite. It can be hard for people to change and some people are just blissfully unaware. Be happy in the knowledge that you're making a difference and try to feel compassionate to people no matter what choices they make. If you are content with who you are, it is more likely that people will be open to talking to you about this. They could even begin questioning their own choices. I have known so many people that have gotten upset and hurt when vegans challenged them and pushed too far. But by simply being an awesome and secure person who's happy in their choices, you'll probably begin to see that your friends want to come to you because they see you so happy and want to know what your secret is.

Finding new items and recipes can be a fun and exciting adventure and a great way to keep yourself on track. We can always learn new things and for a lot of people, going on little adventures can be a lot of fun. Get out and about and see what vegan things you can find around you.

Find inspiration. There are so many celebrities that have taken up the cause and so many other people as well. Doctors, lawyers, teachers; there are so many people now that have joined the vegan move. There are also many organizations that have taken up the movement as well. Be careful with these organizations though and make sure they are on the up and up. Studies have shown that some organizations kill more animals than they save. Or some don't follow the ideas you have for yourself. You need to make sure that you find inspiration that is going to help you. Thanks to social media, you can even be connected to hundreds of thousands of people that have the same lifestyle and desire to help animals as you do. You can ask questions and learn everything you can about the vegan lifestyle. As with anything on social media though, you need to be careful as there are dangers beyond bad advice as some people simply can't be trusted so you'll need to be careful that you don't get hurt.

Grow your own food. This one not everyone can do. Obviously, if you live in an apartment or are renting a house, you have to follow rules and wouldn't be able to do this one. But if you can, grow your own food. You could grow the food you eat and earn a deeper appreciation for your food and what's going in your body. You'll be able to see the work and effort it takes to provide yourself sustenance and you might even help other people try new things because the tastes are different. You can grow anything from vegetables to spices. The really cool thing though is if there's something you want to eat but can't find it anywhere, you can grow it yourself. Now, obviously, if you have to grow it, you won't get it when you want it because it would take weeks or months before it would be ready to eat. However, you will be able to have access to it which is a pretty cool thing to think about. If your garden got big enough, you could share with your finds and family and maybe they would be interested in eating healthier foods for themselves and their family because of your example.

Another surprising thing in this digital age is that you can have groceries delivered to you, even fresh ones in certain cases. This might help people who don't have vegan options near them. It will be easier for you to have it delivered especially if you live far away from the city or you're far from a place that actually carries what you need. Online shopping can also be a great way to try some new snacks as long as you're making sure it's not junk food or overly processed stuff that is going to make you gain a lot of weight. Look for options you know are good.

Remember, this is a journey. If you slip up, forgive and motivate yourself to do better so it won't happen again. If you're tired of the current options you're eating, find/keep trying new recipes and foods that you love. Keep looking around and exploring so that your knowledge keeps expanding. This can be a really fun way to make yourself happy and healthy and make sure that you accomplish the goals that you want to reach for yourself.

Chapter 8 Vegan meal plan

Week 1

Shopping List

- 2 kiwis
- 3 packages of spinach
- 1 kale
- 24 bananas
- 1 package of spelt flour
- 3 packages of ground flaxseeds
- 1 package of salt
- 2 packages of cinnamon
- 1 package of almonds
- 3 packages of hazelnuts
- 2 packages of walnuts
- 2 packages of pecans
- 1 package of dried fruit (of choice)
- 2 packages of vanilla extract
- 1 package of couscous
- 1 bottle of maple syrup
- 1 bottle of olive oil
- 3 packages of chickpeas
- 18 onions
- 1 package of cumin
- 1 package of turmeric
- 2 red peppers
- 8 sweet potatoes
- 1 package of ground coriander
- 2 packages of vegetable stock
- 11 carrots
- 1 package of cayenne pepper
- 2 packages of cilantro
- 4 lemons

- 2 cans full fat coconut milk
- 3 packages of coconut milk
- 2 packages of phylum husk
- 1 package of raspberries
- 2 packages of black beans
- 1 package of kidney beans
- 14 tomatoes
- 1 bottle of stevia
- 1 package of black pepper
- 2 packages of mushrooms
- 1 package of chili powder
- 1 package of oregano
- 1 package of thyme
- 1 package of bay leaves
- 1 can of sweet corn
- 1 bottle of lime juice
- 11 red bell peppers
- 1 peach
- 2 mangos
- 1 orange
- 1 pineapple
- 3 packages of blueberries
- 2 coconuts
- 2 packages of rolled oats
- 2 packages of coconut flour
- 2 packages of almond flour
- 1 package of red lentils
- 1 package of coconut flakes (unsweetened)
- 3 packages of hemp seeds
- 1 package of chia seeds
- 2 packages of almond milk
- 1 package of coconut oil
- 1 ginger root
- 1 package of spicy paprika powder

- 5 heads of garlic
- 1 package of tabasco sauce
- 1 bottle of MCT oil
- 1 eggplant
- 1 package of tahini
- 1 bottle of flaxseed oil
- 1 packages of baking powder
- 3 packages of coconut cream
- 1 package of cocoa powder
- 3 packages of tempeh
- 1 purple cabbage
- 2 packages of quinoa
- 1 package of soy sauce
- 1 bottle of sesame oil
- 1 bottle of rice vinegar
- 1 package of chili flakes
- 1 package of red curry paste
- 2 packages of cashews
- 2 packages of nutritional yeast
- 1 package of paprika powder
- 1 bottle of red wine
- 10 potatoes
- 2 fresh parsleys
- 3 celery stalks
- 1 package of miso
- 1 papaya
- 1 yellow bell pepper
- 1 package of frozen greens (i.e. spinach, kale)
- 1 package of mixed frozen berries
- 2 sweet onions
- 1 package of whole wheat flour
- 1 package of smoked paprika powder
- 1 brown bread
- 1 package of green chili flakes

- 1 package of coconut butter
- 1 package of firm tofu
- 2 packages of brown rice
- 1 radish
- 1 cucumber
- 1 package of edamame(shelled)
- 1 package of sesame seeds
- 1 package of cocoa butter
- 1 package of vegan protein powder
- 1 package of dried thyme
- 1 package of broccoli
- 1 package of nutmeg
- 1 package of basil

Week 2

Shopping List

- 16 bananas
- 3 packages of coconut milk
- 2 packages of blueberries
- 2 packages of raspberries
- 2 packages of vanilla extract
- 3 packages of rolled oats
- 1 package of walnuts
- 2 packages of chia seeds
- 3 packages of black beans
- 4 heads of garlic
- 1 sweet onion
- 3 green bell peppers
- 2 packages of whole wheat flour
- 2 packages of smoked paprika powder
- 1 package of cumin
- 1 package of salt
- 1 package of pepper
- 1 brown bread
- 6 tortillas (whole wheat)
- 3 packages of tempeh
- 3 packages of quinoa
- 7 red bell peppers
- 1 purple cabbage
- 2 sweet potatoes
- 1 kale
- 1 package of broccoli
- 1 bottle of sesame oil
- 1 bottle of soy sauce
- 1 bottle of rice vinegar
- 1 bottle of stevia

- 2 packages of brown rice
- 2 dark vegan chocolates
- 1 package of vanilla flavored vegan protein powder
- 2 kiwis
- 2 packages of spinach
- 2 packages of ground flaxseeds
- 1 pineapple
- 1 mango
- 1 bottle of flaxseed oil
- 1 bottle of olive oil
- 3 packages of hemp seeds
- 2 packages of almond flour
- 3 packages of baking powder
- 7 red onions
- 6 sweet red peppers
- 2 cans (4oz) of green chilis
- 1 package of dry pinto beans
- 1 package of white beans
- 1 package of kidney beans
- 1 roma tomato
- 1 package of paprika powder
- 3 fresh cilantros
- 1 avocado
- 1 package of cilantro
- 1 ginger root
- 3 green onions
- 4 zucchinis
- 1 package of sesame seeds
- 1 jar of peanut butter
- 1 package of chili flakes
- 1 bottle of maple syrup
- 1 package of almonds
- 1 package of pumpkin seeds
- 1 package of dates

- 1 vanilla stick
- 1 bottle of agave nectar
- 3 packages of almond milk
- 1 package of cinnamon
- 1 package of cayenne pepper
- 3 jalapeno peppers
- 1 yellow squash
- 1 bottle of tomato paste
- 2 cans of sweet corn
- 1 package of chili powder
- 1 coconut
- 1 bottle of MCT oil
- 3 packages of cashews
- 1 lime
- 1 package of oat milk
- 1 package of coconut oil
- 1 package of kosher salt
- 1 package of whole wheat spaghetti
- 1 package of tahini
- 2 lemons
- 1 package of Dijon mustard
- 1 package of nutritional yeast
- 1 package of sweet paprika powder
- 1 package of nutmeg
- 1 package of asparagus
- 1 package of peas
- 1 package of baking soda
- 1 package of chickpeas
- 1 package of spicy paprika powder
- 1 package of baby spinach
- 1 package of oregano
- 1 package of avocado oil
- 1 package of garlic powder
- 1 bottle of canola oil

Week 3

Shopping List

- 1 package of rolled oats
- 1 package of oat milk
- 1 package of coconut oil
- 3 packages of ground flaxseeds
- 1 package of chia seeds
- 1 package of vanilla sticks
- 1 package of kosher salt
- 1 package of cinnamon
- 1 package of psyllium husk
- 2 cans of full fat coconut milk
- 1 bottle of stevia
- 5 lemons
- 3 packages of raspberries
- 1 bottle of olive oil
- 3 packages of black beans
- 5 green onions
- 6 red bell peppers
- 1 package of mushrooms
- 1 package of cumin
- 1 package of tabasco sauce
- 1 package of chili powder
- 1 package of salt
- 1 package of sugar
- 2 packages of whole wheat flour
- 1 package of coconut oil
- 1 package of almond butter
- 1 package of almond flour
- 4 packages of almond milk
- 1 bottle of sesame oil

- 2 packages of tofu (1 extra firm)
- 2 packages of baking soda
- 1 package of sesame seeds
- 3 zucchinis
- 1 package of almonds
- 1 package of coconut flour
- 2 packages of oatmeal
- 13 bananas
- 2 packages of hemp seeds
- 1 package of lentils
- 1 ginger root
- 9 onions (2 yellow onions)
- 1 head of garlic
- 1 package of tomato paste
- 1 package of curry powder
- 1 package of red hot pepper flakes
- 1 jar of diced tomatoes
- 1 package of pepper
- 2 cilantros
- 2 packages of spinach
- 2 kales
- 14 carrots
- 6 celery stalks
- 1 package of nutritional yeast
- 1 package of thyme
- 4 fresh parsleys
- 1 package of vanilla flavored vegan protein powder
- 1 dark vegan chocolate
- 1 bottle of MCT oil
- 1 package of cocoa powder
- 1 package of brown rice
- 1 package of white rice
- 1 package of hazelnut
- 1 package of hazelnut spread

- 1 package of vanilla extract
- 1 can of sweet corn
- 2 packages of quinoa
- 1 tomato
- 6 sweet potatoes
- 1 green bell pepper
- 1 lime
- 2 packages of blueberries
- 1 package of strawberries
- 1 package of blackberries
- 1 bag(300g) of tortilla chips
- 4 large tortillas (whole wheat)

Week 4

Shopping list

- 2 green apples
- 1 package of sea salt
- 1 package of red pepper flakes
- 1 bottle of cherry vinegar
- 1 package of black pepper
- 1 package of miso
- 1 package of rosemary
- 2 packages of baking powder
- 1 pumpkin
- 1 package of dark chocolate chips (vegan friendly)
- 4 jazz apples
- 4 Red Delicious apples
- 15 oz of tempeh
- 1 purple cabbage
- 1 package of broccoli
- 1 package of soy sauce
- 1 bottle of rice vinegar
- 2 packages of cashews
- 1 package of chili flakes
- 1 package of red curry paste
- 2 packages of coconut milk
- 2 packages of coconut cream
- 1 kiwi
- 2 apples
- 1 pineapple
- 1 mango
- 1 package of couscous
- 1 package of chickpeas
- 1 red pepper
- 1 package of cayenne pepper

- 1 package of cilantro
- 1 package of coriander
- 1 package of ground turmeric
- 2 packages of vegetable stock
- 1 bottle of avocado oil
- 1 package of garlic powder
- 1 package of oregano
- 3 Chioggia beets
- 2 avocados
- 1 package of wasabi powder
- 1 package of sushi rice
- 2 packages of edamame beans
- 1 package of pecans
- 1 package of matcha powder
- 1 package of freeze dried peach powder
- 1 eggplant
- 1 package of tahini
- 1 package of coconut butter
- 1 package of sriracha
- 1 package of brown sugar
- 1 package of wasabi paste
- 1 package of pickled ginger

Chapter 9: Diet plan

Just knowing the recipes is not good enough. You must have a plan of what and when to eat. Many people who are new to the vegan lifestyle will probably have trouble coming up with a diet plan. Now, I am going to suggest a simple vegan diet plan. Try it. It really works. Since you are changing your diet altogether, the first week of the new diet plan can have more calories, so that your body gets used to reduce in the amount of calories and fats slowly. The 4-week diet plan is based on less than 1200 calories a day (similar to a typical vegan diet). The amount of food from this may be inadequate, usually for men and very active individuals. If you fit into these categories, you will most likely lose weight. As I have mentioned earlier, the diet can be flexibly changed based on the person. Ask your dietitian about your normal calorie intake and modify the plan accordingly.

Week 1

Monday

Breakfast: Keto Porridge
Lunch: Cauliflower Coconut Rice
Dinner: Asian Cucumber Salad
Dessert: Avocado Pudding

Tuesday

Breakfast: Easy Chia Seed Pudding
Lunch: Fried Okra
Dinner: Mexican Cauliflower Rice
Dessert: Almond Butter Brownies

Wednesday

Breakfast: Delicious Vegan Zoodles
Lunch: Asparagus Mash
Dinner: Turnip Salad
Dessert: Raspberry Chia Pudding

Thursday

Breakfast: Avocado Tofu Scramble
Lunch: Baked Asparagus

Dinner: Brussels sprouts Salad
Dessert: Chocolate Fudge

Friday

Breakfast: Delicious Tofu Fries
Lunch: Spinach with Coconut Milk

Dinner: Tomato Eggplant Spinach Salad

Dessert: Quick Chocó Brownie

Saturday

Breakfast: Chia Raspberry Pudding Shots
Lunch: Delicious Cabbage Steaks

Dinner: Cauliflower Radish Salad

Dessert: Simple Almond Butter Fudge

Sunday

Breakfast: Healthy Chia-Almond Pudding

Lunch: Tomato Avocado Cucumber Salad
Dinner: Cabbage Coconut Salad
Dessert: Coconut Peanut Butter Fudge

For the first week, since you are still trying to get used to a new lifestyle and totally new diet, I recommend these food items with calorific value so as to not throw off your body and keep it in balance and also you won't feel that hungry and give up in the first week itself.

Sunday's breakfast can be taken lightly as you can have more calories in the other meals of the day. I chose Sunday because, it is the only day you won't need much energy in the morning. But for people who work on Sunday too, you can change the food menu but make sure you balance it out with consuming fewer amounts of calories in your other meals. And remember, breakfast is the most important meal of the day, therefore do not skip it. Keep in mind that smoothies can be a great option for breakfast too.

Week 2

Let us start reducing the intake of calories gradually.

Monday

Breakfast: Fresh Berries with Cream
Lunch: Tomato Avocado Cucumber Salad

Dinner: Cabbage Coconut Salad

Dessert: Coconut Peanut Butter Fudge

Tuesday

Breakfast: Almond Hemp Heart Porridge
Lunch: Tomato Avocado Cucumber Salad
Dinner: Cabbage Coconut Salad
Dessert: Coconut Peanut Butter Fudge

Wednesday

Breakfast: Almond Hemp Heart Porridge
Lunch: Tomato Avocado Cucumber Salad
Dinner: Cabbage Coconut Salad
Dessert: Coconut Peanut Butter Fudge

Thursday

Breakfast: Cauliflower Zucchini Fritters
Lunch: Tomato Avocado Cucumber Salad
Dinner: Cabbage Coconut Salad
Dessert: Coconut Peanut Butter Fudge

Friday

Breakfast: Chocolate Strawberry Milkshake
Lunch: Tomato Avocado Cucumber Salad

Dinner: Cabbage Coconut Salad
Dessert: Coconut Peanut Butter Fudge

Saturday

Breakfast: Coconut Blackberry Breakfast Bowl
Lunch: Tomato Avocado Cucumber Salad
Dinner: Cabbage Coconut Salad
Dessert: Coconut Peanut Butter Fudge

Sunday

Breakfast: Cinnamon Coconut Pancake
Lunch: Tomato Avocado Cucumber Salad
Dinner: Cabbage Coconut Salad
Dessert: Coconut Peanut Butter Fudge

I have recommended the desserts with more calories, because desserts generally tend to make you slow. So, it's better to have them in weekends rather than during the weekdays when you have to work hard.

Week 3

From this week on, the calories that you are going to consume are going to go down by a great extent. The calorie levels in all the meals will be very little. So make sure you adjust whatever you want to, to get the right combination and make sure that you get enough calories required for your body to function.

Monday

Breakfast: Flax Almond Muffins
Lunch: Tomato Avocado Cucumber Salad
Dinner: Cabbage Coconut Salad
Dessert: Coconut Peanut Butter Fudge

Tuesday

Breakfast: Grain-free Overnight Oats
Lunch: Tomato Avocado Cucumber Salad
Dinner: Cabbage Coconut Salad
Dessert: Coconut Peanut Butter Fudge

Wednesday

Breakfast: Apple Avocado Coconut Smoothie
Lunch: Tomato Avocado Cucumber Salad

Dinner: Cabbage Coconut Salad
Dessert: Coconut Peanut Butter Fudge

Thursday

Breakfast: Chia Cinnamon Smoothie
Lunch: Tomato Avocado Cucumber Salad
Dinner: Cabbage Coconut Salad
Dessert: Coconut Peanut Butter Fudge

Friday

Breakfast: Vegetable Tofu Scramble
Lunch: Tomato Avocado Cucumber Salad
Dinner: Cabbage Coconut Salad
Dessert: Coconut Peanut Butter Fudge

Saturday

Breakfast: Strawberry Chia Matcha Pudding
Lunch: Tomato Avocado Cucumber Salad
Dinner: Cabbage Coconut Salad
Dessert: Coconut Peanut Butter Fudge

Sunday

Breakfast: Healthy Spinach Green Smoothie

Lunch: Tomato Avocado Cucumber Salad

Dinner: Cabbage Coconut Salad

Dessert: Coconut Peanut Butter Fudge

Week 4

Since this is the last week, the calorie intake is meager. Let's have a look at it.

Monday

Breakfast: Fresh Berries with Cream
Lunch: Tomato Avocado Cucumber Salad
Dinner: Cabbage Coconut Salad
Dessert: Coconut Peanut Butter Fudge

Tuesday

Breakfast: Avocado Breakfast Smoothie
Lunch: Tomato Avocado Cucumber Salad
Dinner: Cabbage Coconut Salad
Dessert: Coconut Peanut Butter Fudge

Wednesday

Breakfast: Almond Coconut Porridge
Lunch: Tomato Avocado Cucumber Salad
Dinner: Cabbage Coconut Salad
Dessert: Coconut Peanut Butter Fudge

Thursday

Breakfast: *Cinnamon* Muffin
Lunch: Tomato Avocado Cucumber Salad
Dinner: Cabbage Coconut Salad
Dessert: Coconut Peanut Butter Fudge

Friday

Breakfast: Cinnamon Muffin
Lunch: Tomato Avocado Cucumber Salad
Dinner: Cabbage Coconut Salad
Dessert: Coconut Peanut Butter Fudge

Saturday

Breakfast: Cauliflower Zucchini Fritters
Lunch: Tomato Avocado Cucumber Salad
Dinner: Cabbage Coconut Salad
Dessert: Coconut Peanut Butter Fudge

Sunday

Breakfast: Flax Almond Muffins
Lunch: Tomato Avocado Cucumber Salad
Dinner: Cabbage Coconut Salad
Dessert: Coconut Peanut Butter Fudge

I am recommending this kind of a diet plan, because after this, you will become used to every situation. You will be eating very well during the first week, and then gradually reducing the calorie levels and then almost to nothing. This way you will be prepared to whatever routine you want to follow. Once you do this, you will exactly know how much calories your body requires to function normally and choose your diet plan accordingly.

Conclusion

A vegan diet will bring you so many amazing benefits and it will improve your overall health. The vegan diet is easy to follow as long as you respect its principles. If you are going to embrace this diet, you should really take a look at this great guide. You will learn how to prepare the best vegan breakfasts, soups, salads, main dishes, and desserts. Does this sound great of what?

So, get your hands on this great collection and start making some of the best vegan dishes for you and all your loved ones. Start a vegan diet now and enjoy the cooking guide you just discovered. Savor each dish gathered in this collection and find out how amazing it is to be on a vegan diet.

Is the vegan diet healthy enough?

The vegan diet makes you healthier, fitter, and stronger. But similarly to any diet, it is only as good as its follower. If you only consume meals full of trans fats, preservatives, or sodium, and regularly drink sugary beverages, then your diet is unhealthy. However, forgoing all the unhealthy options above and applying the clean eating techniques in this book guarantees health improvements.

Nutritional benefits of vegan food

Low saturated fats: are excellent for your heart.

- High fibers: provide better digestive health, lower sugar cravings, and protect against certain cancers.

- Increased magnesium: aids calcium absorption thus improving bone health.

- *High antioxidant levels:* remove free radicals and protects against cellular damage.
- Increased potassium: maintains PH levels, lowers acidity, and stimulates kidney function.

Disease Prevention

- *Whole grains and nuts:* reduce the risk of Type-2 diabetes, gallstones, hypertension, and certain cancers.
- *Vegetables and fruits:* prevent macular degeneration.

Physical Benefits

- Healthy fats: help lose weight and boost energy levels.
- Vitamins in vegetables and nuts: improve skin and hair health.

Eliminating animal foods can also reduce body odor and bad breath.

CPSIA information can be obtained
at www.ICGtesting.com
Printed in the USA
LVHW060815260621
690828LV00019B/277

9 789820 6947